Cytohormonal Profile of a Female

from Birth to Postmenopausal Phase

A Review

Cytohormonal Profile of a Female
from Birth to Postmenopausal Phase

A Review

Ansar Abbas Khan

MBBS, MD Pathology (India), C Cytol (UK)

Retired Professor
Department of Pathology
Jawaharlal Nehru Medical College
Aligarh Muslim University
Aligarh, India

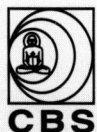

CBS

CBS Publishers & Distributors Pvt Ltd

New Delhi • Bengaluru • Chennai • Kochi • Kolkata • Mumbai
Hyderabad • Nagpur • Patna • Pune

Cytohormonal Profile of a Female
from Birth to Postmenopausal Phase

A Review

ISBN: 978-93-86478-09-2

First Edition: 2017

Published by Satish Kumar Jain and produced by Varun Jain for

CBS Publishers & Distributors Pvt Ltd

4819/XI Prahlad Street, 24 Ansari Road, Daryaganj, New Delhi 110 002, India.
Ph: 23289259, 23266861, 23266867   Website: www.cbspd.com
Fax: 011-23243014   e-mail: delhi@cbspd.com; cbspubs@airtelmail.in.

Corporate Office: 204 FIE, Industrial Area, Patparganj, Delhi 110 092
Ph: 4934 4934   Fax: 4934 4935   e-mail: publishing@cbspd.com; publicity@cbspd.com

Branches

- **Bengaluru:** Seema House 2975, 17th Cross, K.R. Road,
  Banasankari 2nd Stage, Bengaluru 560 070, Karnataka
  Ph: +91-80-26771678/79   Fax: +91-80-26771680   e-mail: bangalore@cbspd.com
- **Chennai:** 7, Subbaraya Street, Shenoy Nagar, Chennai 600 030, Tamil Nadu
  Ph: +91-44-26680620, 26681266   Fax: +91-44-42032115   e-mail: chennai@cbspd.com
- **Kochi:** Ashana House, No. 39/1904, AM Thomas Road, Valanjambalam,
  Ernakulam 682 016, Kochi, Kerala
  Ph: +91-484-4059061-62-64-65   Fax: +91-484-4059065   e-mail: kochi@cbspd.com
- **Kolkata:** 6/B, Ground Floor, Rameswar Shaw Road, Kolkata-700 014, West Bengal
  Ph: +91-33-22891126, 22891127, 22891128   e-mail: kolkata@cbspd.com
- **Mumbai:** 83-C, Dr E Moses Road, Worli, Mumbai-400018, Maharashtra
  Ph: +91-22-24902340/41   Fax: +91-22-24902342   e-mail: mumbai@cbspd.com

Representatives

- **Hyderabad** 0-9885175004   • **Nagpur** 0-9021734563
- **Patna**   0-9334159340   • **Pune**   0-9623451994

Printed at: Rashtriya Printers, Dilshad Garden, Delhi, India

to
_____

the memory of my mother
Ayesha Begum

Foreword

It gives me great pleasure to write the Foreword for this very interesting book on hormonal cytology.

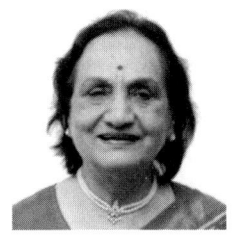

The author and I have been involved in cytology now for over half a century. We have seen the introduction of vaginal cytology in the diagnostic armamentarium of the gynecologist. We have witnessed the "revolution" caused by pap smear which brought down the incidence and mortality of invasive cervical cancer in some parts of the world.

We also learned to use simple techniques like the cervical mucus test and vaginal cytology to sort out hormonal disorders such as amenorrhoea and infertility.

However, since these early days much water has flown down the rivers. Technology has advanced rapidly with the availability of ultrasound scans and radioimmunoassays of all hormones available freely. The need to depend on cytology has greatly diminished.

Certain other issues have also made us understand that it is not just the blood levels of circulating of hormones which are reflected in the cellular pattern. Tissue receptors and their functionality, bioavailability of hormones and the diagnosis of cell metabolism are all important players. Finally, it is the end organ response which will need to be addressed to and treated. Herein lies the innate value of cytology which alone indicates the end organ response.

The author has dealt in detail with all the patterns seen in health and disease. The writing and diagrams are simple to follow and will certainly provide a clinician an insight into the world of cellular response.

Phase contrast microscopy is a new tool in the hands of a clinician. This simple equipment enables a gynecologist to study a "hanging drop" specimen of cervicovaginal fluid to know the dynamic changes going on in the epithelium. Without any laboratory support, staining, fixing, etc., the floating cells and the organism can be noted and diagnosis is available in five minutes. This chapter written by a world renowned scientist in phase contrast microscopy will open up a new vista for the younger generations of clinicians who believe in evidence-based medicine.

This publication has great historic value. A diagnostic tool widely used for over 50 years, which enabled the development of the superspecialty of endocrinology, needed to be chronicled for posterity. We must all congratulate the author Dr Ansar Khan for undertaking and completing this gigantic task.

And to all the readers, I wish them good luck and enjoyable reading. In this era of information technology this whole world of hormonal cytology will be available to everyone all over the world at the click of a mouse. This is truly a miracle of the 21st century.

With warm personal regards and best wishes to all who made this publication a reality.

Dr Usha Saraiya

Founder Member and President (1984-86), Indian Academy of Cytologists
President, Mumbai Obst. and Gyn. Society (1997-1998)
President, Federation of Obstetrics and Gynaecological Societies of India (2002)
Chairman, Indian College of Obstetrics and Gynaecology (2006-2009)
Awarded Outstanding Women Obstetrician Gynaecologist Award of FIGO (2003)
Pandit Award of MOGS for outstanding contribution to Women's Empowerment (2014)
Dr BN Purandare outstanding Services Award by MOGS in January (2015)

Currently

Chairman, Ethics Committee for Clinical Research of National Institute for Research in Reproductive Health, ICMR
Vice President, Medical Women's International Association
Trustee, Mumbai Obstetric and Gynaecological Society (MOGS)

Acknowledgements

It is with a deep sense of personal gratitude that I wish to thank Dr Usha Saraiya for providing her published work on some aspects of endocrine cytology and the contribution of literature along with the microphotographs of her patients on phase contrast direct microscopy.

I am oblidged to Dr Rashmi Hegde, MD, DCh, who helped me in getting the manuscript edited, without which I could not have completed this book.

Many thanks are due to Dr Shamim Jahan Rizvi, who allowed me to publish the data of her research, carried out under my guidance in 1975–76. She has recently retired as Professor and Chairperson, Department of Forensic Medicine, JNMC, AMU, Aligarh, UP.

I wish to express my gratitude to Dr Ruqqia Rizvi, retired gynaecologist, JNMC, AMU, Aligarh, UP, for her generous help in providing the material for research and routine work.

I am indebted to my son, Mr Rehan Abbas Khan, President, Asia Pacific, DaVita, who gave me continuous encouragement and moral support, while I was writing this book.

I would like to record my appreciation for the technical staff Mr Sayeed Ahmad, Mrs Neelofer Gani and Mr Chand Mohd for the help in laboratory work for over three decades, while I was working at JNMC, Aligarh.

I am thankful to Mr Azad who performed the preliminary formatting of this book and Mrs Sunita Gehani, who finally edited it with personal care.

I would be failing in my duty, if I do not thank Mrs Nusrat Shariff, Nighat Abbas, Dr Kafil Akhter and Zia Ur Rehman Khan for their help in the compilation of this book for publication.

Ansar A Khan

Contents

Introduction

Virchow first put forward the concept of cellular pathology which Papanicolaou introduced in laboratory medicine after studying an unstained vaginal smear of a pregnant female under the microscope (1925).

In modern research and in special cases in gynecological practice, the studies of hormonal (exfoliative) cytology can be carried out with the help of newer advanced techniques such as flow cytometry, cytochemistry, the florescent technique, the phase contrast and electron microscopy, all of which require a well established, sophisticated laboratory as found only in big cities. These newer techniques are expensive and it is not the privilege of the common man in day-to-day practice in India.

Exfoliative cytology is now a well accepted technique all over the world in routine practice, as it is easy, simple, cheap and reliable. Further it is a non-surgical and atraumatic quick diagnostic tool; hence easily accepted by a female patient for the assessment of her hormonal status as well as for detection of cancer, particularly in cases of the cancer cervix uteri. Exfoliative cytology studies have proved that early diagnosis of pre-cancerous lesions and carcinoma *in situ* of the cervix uteri, have allowed cure of up to 100% in these cases.

Prof PN Wahi, one of the pioneer workers of India in the field of cytopathology, introduced it in clinical practice in SN Medical College, Agra, India, in 1950. In his address at the first seminar in India on exfoliative cytology in 1969, organized by Indian Council of Medical Research (ICMR), Prof Wahi mentioned that to gain acceptance, every laboratory technique has to fulfill the following criteria:

1. Diagnostic accuracy
2. Simplicity in performance
3. Avoidance of discomfort to the patient

Exfoliative cytology has not only fulfilled the above criteria but has also revealed the additional advantages over the old and classical technique of biopsy, that in addition to being a quick, safe, reliable, economical, and atraumatic technique, it can be repeated as many times as desired. Further, it does not require hospitalization and can be performed in the outpatient department of a hospital as well as in an office of a private clinic.

Exfoliative cytology is a branch of life sciences, which deals with the study of morphological and functional changes in each cell, shed off in the body cavities. It is utilized for providing a dynamic insight into the hormonal changes in a female from birth to the post-menopausal phases as well as for diagnosis of cancer in male and female subjects.

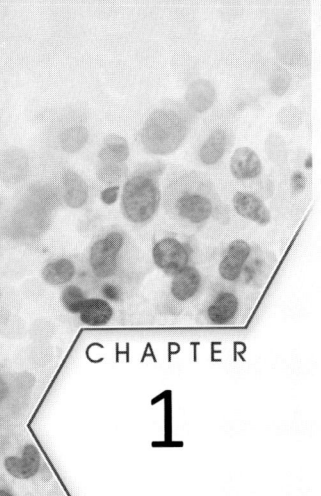

History of Endocrine Cytology

The early attempts at cytodiagnosis in the field of Endocrine Cytology appeared in the form of Pauchet's monograph (1847). After a long period of fifty years, Papanicolaou in 1925 published his first report of a smear of the vaginal secretion of a pregnant woman, in which he found the boat shaped cells (now known as navicular cells) which he, at that time, thought were diagnostic of early pregnancy.

In the next two decades the technique of exfoliative cytology was mainly utilized for the diagnosis of cancer of the female genital tract, particularly the cancer cervix uteri.

Shorr in 1941 introduced a polychrome stain for the endocrine cytology smear, which only stained the cytoplasm of the cell. Later, in 1942, Papanicolaou discovered another polychrome stain which not only stained the cytoplasm but the nuclear DNA also. Both these stains give a spectrum of colour to the cytoplasm, that is, blue, green, pink, and orange, indicating the effect of hormones, which are responsible for the different stages of maturity of the cells.Traut in 1943 slightly modified this stain but it still goes by the name of Papanicolaou, as Pap. stain.

Later some American workers, Papanicolaou (1936), Rubenstein (1940), Neustaedter (1944) and Brown (1949) published their reports on the cellular contents of the vaginal smears, which constituted an approximate gauge of the oestrogen activity of the vaginal cells. European workers Gaudefroy and Van Meensel (1950) introduced some numerical criteria for the evaluation of vaginal cytology. Pundal (1950) published comparative cell studies, based on Karyopyknotic and eosinophilic indices. After this, Nyklicek (1951) introduced a cytogram, which was later developed into the maturation index of Frost,who presented it at the Terminology Symposium in 1958. All the indices as a cumulative index related to estimation of oestrogen level were called as "Oestrogen Value" by Meisels till 1966.

Schmitt (1953) published a numerical pattern of the degrees of cell maturity which was amplified by Wied in 1955 to encompass the criteria of cell folding and crowding in vaginal cells, while Langreder in 1953 used a rather cumbersome cytometry for cell classification. In 1958 Wied, delSol and Dargan suggested that the crowded cell index (CCI) and folded cell index (FCI), could be used as additional records of cell criteria for studying the progesterone effect in the vaginal smear.

Meisels (1967), after a discussion in the tutorial on hormonal cytology (organized by Wied) suggested that the "Oestrogen value", based on Karyopyknotic Index, Eosinophilic Index and Maturation Index, should be replaced by the "Maturation Value" of Frost, which is a cumulative value of cell maturity and it accurately describes the phenomenon which one wants to measure with this value. With the increased application of computers, the index, Maturation Value was subsequently utilized for record keeping and data retrieval of large numbers of patients.

With the introduction of objective criteria in addition to the subjective evaluation of vaginal cytology, these values could then be applied for the study of the various phases of the menstrual cycle, different trimesters of pregnancy and its disorders. The studies allowed the confirmation of the practical value of endocrine cytology not only for diagnostic but for prognostic as well as for therapeutic purposes.

Exfoliative cytology is now a well established and reliable technique for study of the hormonal status of a female. It is found that exfoliative cytology gives results earlier than the hormonal bioassay and chemical analysis; therefore precious time is not wasted in emergencies and treatment is started early.

Recently discovered objective criteria along with the subjective assessment of human observations are the hallmark of diagnostic and prognostic cytopathology and they provide a helpful aid as well as supplement the final diagnosis.

Although cytopathology is based on sound morphological principles, one needs to remember that it cannot be assigned the role of the final arbitrator in every case (Prof. Wahi, 1969).

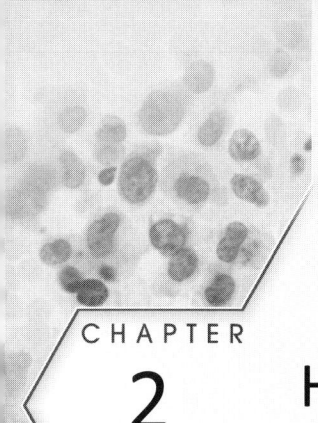

Hypothalamus —Pituitary-Ovary-Uterine Axis

Revision of anatomical and physiological information on the Hypothalamus—Pituitary-Ovary-Uterine Axis is essential in order to understand the hormonal effects on cell cytology. Such a revision is possible through the book B.R. Series–Biology and Histopathology–4th Ed. The Gonadotropin Releasing Hormone (GnRH) from the Neuro Secretory Cells in the Hypothalamus, release stimulating as well as inhibitory hormones (via the feedback from oestrogen and progesterone). Gonadotropin Releasing Hormone regulatesthe release and inhibition of Follicle Stimulating Hormone (FSH) and Luteinising Hormone (LH) from the pituitary via the portal blood vessels as shown in Diagram 2.1.

THE OVARIAN CORTEX

It contains a Large Number of Primordial Follicles

I. **The Primordial Follicle: This** is composed of a Primary Oocyte enveloped by a single layer of flattened follicular cells. This oocyte has a vesicular nucleus with a single nucleolus, and is arrested in the prophase stage of meiosis-I. This remains as such in the foetal life and in the first few years of childhood.

The Primary Follicle: During its development in the reproductive period in the female subject

A. A few out of the many primordial follicles develop into the unilaminar, then multilaminar follicles.

B. These multilaminar follicular cells are now called the granulosa cells which have circumscribed two layers of stromal cells

  a. The inner layer of cells is called the theca interna

  b. The outer fibrous layer is called the theca externa.

  c. These two layers are separated by a layer of basal lamina.

Up to this stage these cells are under the control of the following Paracrine Hormones:

1. Activin

2. Inhibin

3. Folliculostatin (Follistatin)

II. **The Secondary Follicle:**

  a. The liquor in the follicle begins to accumulate into the intercellular spaces between the granulosa cells. These later coalesce to form a large space, called the antrum (A).

  b. These Secondary follicles are under the control of FSH

  c. Granulosa cells secrete Folliculostatin, Inhibin, Activin which along with oestrogen regulate the release of FSH.

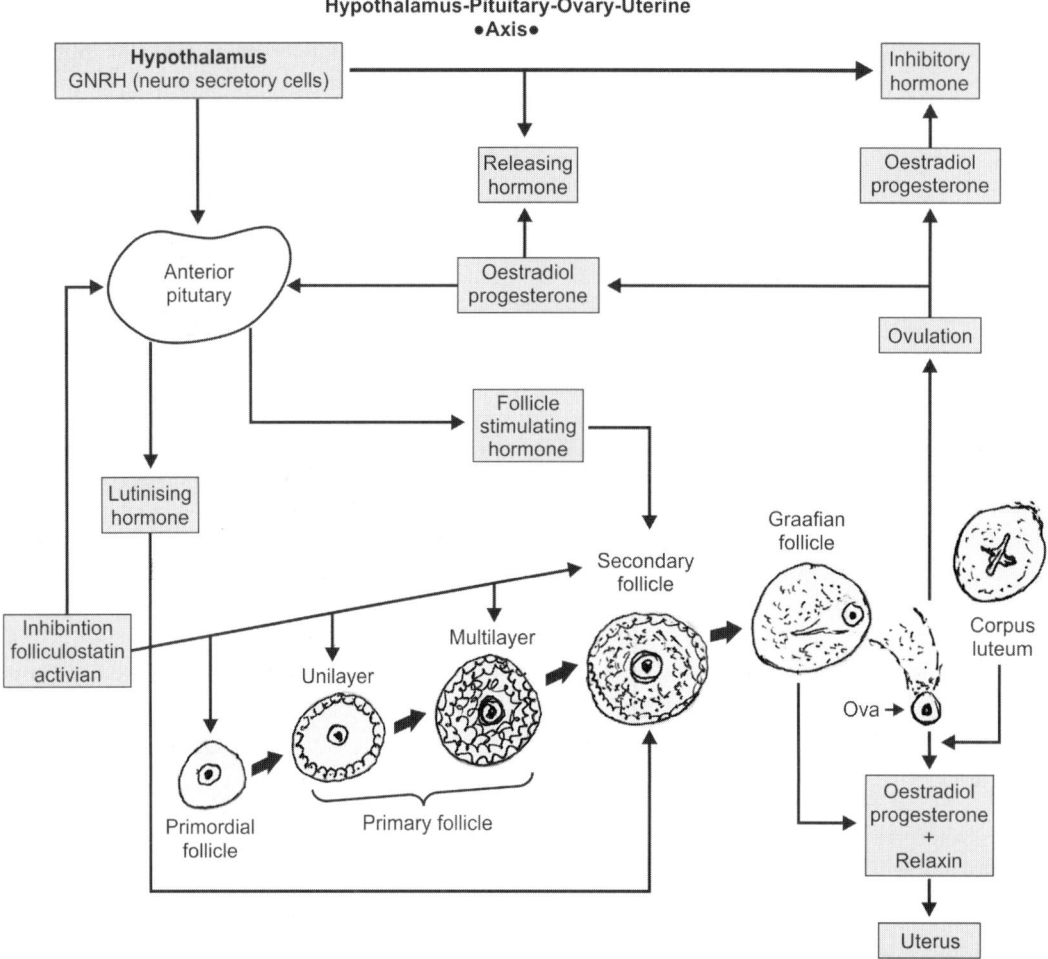

Diagram 2.1: Shows hormonal relationship between the hypophysis and the reproductive system

III. FSH:

i. Stimulates the growth and development of the secondary follicle into a mature follicle.

ii. Theca interna manufactures androgen and transfers it to the granulosa cells. The granulosa cells convert androgen to oestrogen under the effect of FSH.

iii. FSH manufactures the plasmalemma receptors for LH binding

iv. Mature Graafians Follicle is one of the follicles, selected from among the secondary follicles, that will ovulate in a given cycle.

This most mature Graafian Follicle releases its oocyte during ovulation at a time when the oestrogen level is at the highest, approximately on the 14/15th day of the menstrual cycle. The high level of oestrogen, at this time, leads to a brief LH surge.

IV. LH: (Luteinizing Hormone) The brief surge of LH triggers the primary oocyte to complete meiosis I and enter into meiosis II with an arrest at the metaphase stage.

i. LH initiates the process of ovulation of the secondary oocyte from the mature Graafian Follicle.

ii. LH also promotes the formation of the Corpus Luteum.

V. **Corpus Luteum** secretes luteal hormone mainly progesterone in addition to a little amount of oestrogen.

    a. Progesterone dominates and leads to:

      i. Suppression of **Gonadotropin Releasing Hormone,** which inhibits the release of LH,

      ii. It stimulates the proliferation of the endometrium in the uterus.

    b. Oestrogen at its peak secretion, inhibits the release of FSH by suppressing GnRH.

    c. The hormone Relaxin facilitates the parturition action on the uterine tissues.

VI. **In the event of fertilization of the ovum,** the corpus luteum takes up the function of a temporary endocrine gland and maintains pregnancy in the first 3 months (that is, the first trimester of pregnancy). The Corpus Luteum itself is maintained by the hormone Human Chorionic Gonadotrophin (HCG), which is produced by the developing syncytiotrophoblasts of the placenta in the uterus.

After the first trimester (that is, the first 12 weeks of gestation) the placenta completely takes over the function of the corpus luteum to carry on pregnancy until term.

OR

VII. **In the absence of pregnancy**

    a. There is atrophy of the Corpus Luteum leading to withdrawal of the hormones oestrogen and progesterone, which causes menstruation (withdrawal bleeding from the uterus).

    b. The lack of oestrogen and progesterone at the time of the menstruation, stimulates the GnRH and triggers the release of FSH and then LH from the pituitary, and thus reinitiates the "Menstrual Cycle". This cycle is repeated every month during the reproductive period, interrupted by pregnancy, and ceases at menopause.

The ovarian medulla contains large blood vessels, lymphatics and nerves in loose connective tissue stroma. It also contains interstitial cells, which secrete oestrogen and a few hilus cells, which secrete androgen.

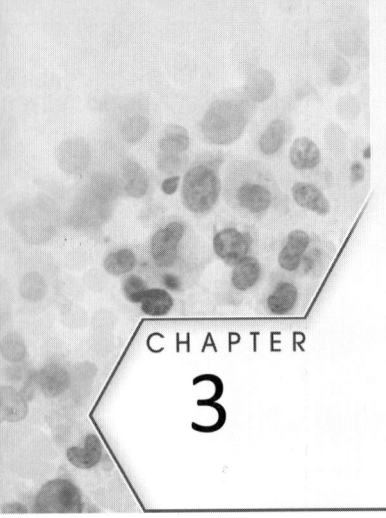

Morphology of Stratified Squamous Epithelium and Exfoliated Cells

Stratified Squamous Epithelium and its Exfoliated Cells : In order to understand the hormonal effects on the vaginal epithelium one is required to study the morphology of the stratified squamous epithelium and the exfoliated cells as shown in Diagram 3.1.

Before The Terminology Symposium of 1958, the assignation of value was as follows:

1. Large eosinopilic polyhedral cells with pyknotic Nucleus = 1.
2. Smaller cyanophilic superficial cell = 0.75.
3. Large cyanophillic intermediate Cell = 0.5.

4. Small cyanophillic intermediate cell. Both show a vesicular nucleus = 0.25
5. Parabasal cells = 0.0 (large vesicular nucleus)

After: The Terminology Symposium of 1958, the large and small cell terminology was discarded and the values assigned to the different cells were as follows:

1. Superficial large and small both eosinophilic and cyanophiliccells, having pyknotic nucleus, were of same value = (one) 1.0.

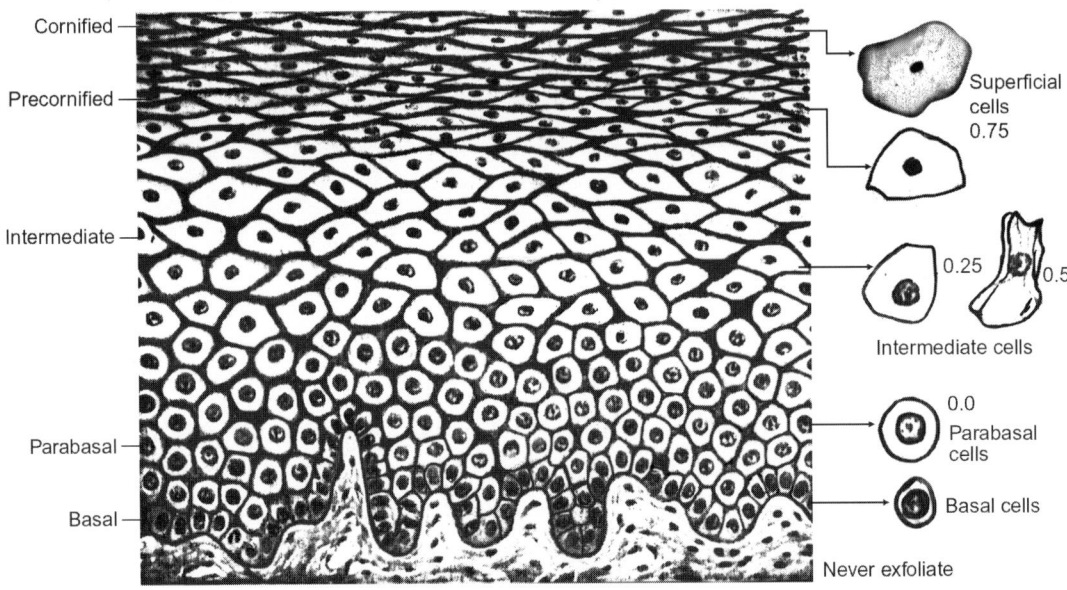

Cornified —
Precornified —
Intermediate —
Parabasal —
Basal —

Superficial cells 0.75

0.25   0.5

Intermediate cells

0.0 Parabasal cells

Basal cells

Never exfoliate

Diagram 3.1

2. Large and small cyanophilic intermediate cells, having vesicular nucleus = 0.5.

3. Parabasal cells = 0.0.

Meisels (1967) suggested that in cases of pregnancy, the intermediate cells should be split as there is a difference in the maturation of small intermediate (**Papanicolaou**'s Navicular cell) andthe large intermediate (Precornified cell). Thus the value to be considered for the small cell would be 0.5 and for the large cell, 0.6.

The epithelial cells of the deepest layer of the stratified squamous epithelium are called the basal cells; these cells do not exfoliate. Above this basal layer is the parabasal cell layer; the cells here are small, round and the most characteristic feature is the large central nucleus occupying most of the cell area and showing a well differentiated chromatin network which stains deeply basophilic. The perinuclear cytoplasm is scanty with light blue staining. These cells are rarely seen in the vaginal smear except in pathological conditions or at puberty and during the post menopausal period.

The intermediate zone cells are large, flat and polygonal with smoothly rounded edges, a homogenous transparent cytoplasm which stains clear blue or violet; the nucleus is centrally placed, large and rounded and it has a well marked chromatin network. Vacuolization in the cytoplasm frequently occurs on account of the glycogen depositions. These show an envelope effect when under the influence of progesterone.

In the superficial zone, the cells are larger, flat and polygonal with pyknotic nuclei. The cytoplasm is clear or occasionally granular which stains pink with Papanicolaou stains, when the pH in the vagina is normal. The criteria of pyknosis for determination of Karyopy knotic Index (KPI) is described by Lukesh (1968), as one of the classical phases of nuclear destruction. There is chromatin condensation with loss of the intranuclear structure and diminution of the nuclear volume. In Haematoxylin and Eosin stain, the nucleus appears as a solid looking blue–black or violet, oval or rounded structure. Its longest diameter should not exceed 6 microns (the size of a small lymphocyte).

The structure of stratified squamous epithelium of the vulva and that of the trigone of the urinary bladder is the same as the vagina.

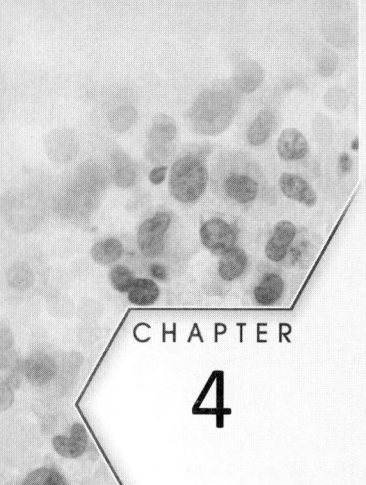

Endocrine Cytology Under the Effect of Hormones

STRATIFIED SQUAMOUS EPITHELIUM

1. Oestrogen Effect

The monohormonal effect of oestrogen on the stratified squamous epithelium is as follows:

  i. Proliferation

 ii. Differentiation

iii. Maturation

  i. **Proliferation:** is the multiplication of cells of each layer; this increase in the number of cells in each layer leads to thickening of the epithelium. It allows heavy exfoliation of all types of cells except basal and parabasal cells under normal conditions. Thus excessive exfoliation of intermediate and superficial cells occurs in different phases of the menstrual cycle as well as in the different trimesters of pregnancy.

 ii. **Differentiation:** In this phase, there is proliferation of one layer of cells into the immediate next layer, that is, from the parabasal cells to the intermediate cells and thereafter the intermediate cyanophilic cells change into the superficial layer. The superficial cells are eosinophilic with pyknotic nuclei. Beyond this, keratinisation of the cytoplasm with dissolution of the nucleus occurs in abnormal conditions only.

iii. **Maturation:** Proliferation and differentiation lead to maturation, which is essentially the shift from the basal to parabasal, then parabasal to the intermediate and from the intermediate to the superficial cells. In this phase, besides this, the size of the cells increases as well as colour of the cytoplasm changes. The deep cyanophilic cytoplasm of the basal layer changes to light blue in the intermediate layer and then to pink or eosinophilic when it reaches the superficial cells. At the same time, the dark, dense, large nucleus of the basal cell becomes cyanophilic and then it turns vesicular in the intermediate cell. In the most mature superficial cell, it is pyknotic and is almost equivalent to the size of a small lymphocyte (5 or 6 microns in diameter).

Most of the superficial exfoliated cells, under the effect of oestrogen are seen clinically in the first half of the menstrual cycle, that is classically, the maximum effect should be seen on the 14/15th day of the menstrual cycle. Ovulation occurs between 12 and 19 days. In the first half of the menstrual cycle, there are mostly large polyhedral superficial cells with transparent eosinophilic cytoplasm and pyknotic nucleus, having sharp borders. This change in the cells is in response to the maturation effect, being the most reliable effect of oestrogen. Previously all these changes were labelled as the oestrogenisation effect; now with the advent of numerical criteria, these effects are measured semi-quantitatively as objective values in the form of the Karyopyknotic index (KPI) and the eosinophilic index (EI). At this stage of oestrogenisation, in the smear, the background is clear, the mucous is elastic, clear and leucopenic. The leucocytes and the micro-organisms (that is, the Deo-derlein bacilli) are not seen. Oestro-genisation measured semiquantitatively as a cumulative effect was previously labelled as "oestrogen value" and was later known as the "Maturation Value", after the Terminology Symposium of 1958.

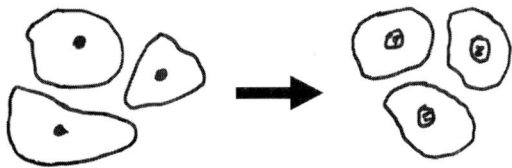

Diagram 4.1: Karyopyknotic index (KPI)

philic staining (regardless of the nuclear appearance) to mature cells with cyanophilic cytoplasm as represented in diagram 4.2.

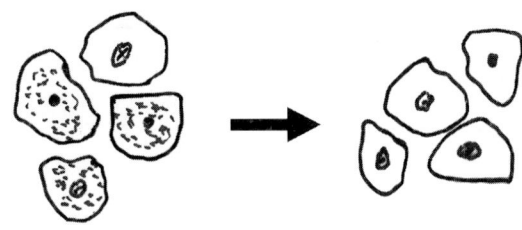

Diagram 4.2: Eosinophilic index (EI)

SEMI QUANTITATIVE ASSESSMENT OF HORMONES

I. Oestrogen

The terminology of indices, described in the symposium on "Hormonal Cytology" (1968) are as follows:

The Karyopyknotic Index: This represents the relation of all mature cells of the squamous epithelium, containing a pyknotic nucleus to the mature squamous cells, containing a vesicular nucleus (regardless of the cyto-plasmic staining of the cells).

Pyknotic Nucleus Size: This should not surpass 6 microns, under high magnification (Cytological Terminology 1958), as shown in diagram 4.1.

The Eosinophilic Index: This index represents the relation of all mature cells with eosino-

The Maturation Index: Nyklicek (1951) introduced the cytogram, which after the "Terminology symposium" of the Inter-national Academy of Cytologists (1958) was changed to "Maturation Index", by Frost (1958). This index represents the relation of the cells-parabasal to intermediate and to superficial, as shown below in Diagram 4.3 (Differential Count) showing M.I.

Superficial Cell Index: The index represents the relation of the superficial mature cells with pyknotic nuclei to all other squamous cells. It is shown in diagram 4.4.

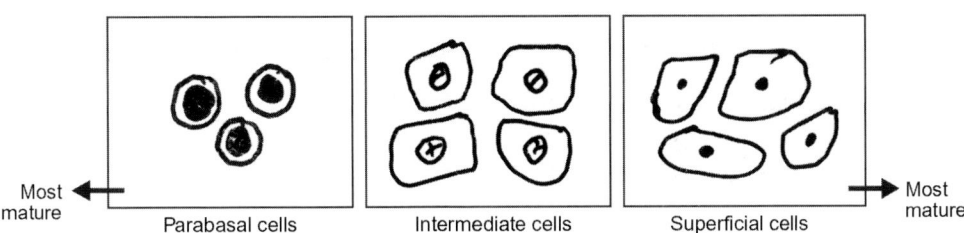

Most mature ← Parabasal cells   Intermediate cells   Superficial cells → Most mature

Diagram 4.3: Maturation index (MI)

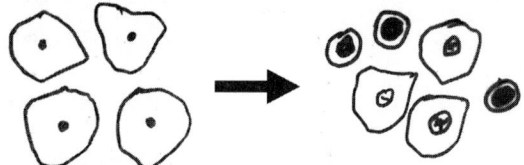

Diagram 4.4: Superficial cell index

The Maturation Value: This index assigns certain values to each cell as shown below. The values of each cell in the differential count are multiplied with the percentage of each cell type. The resultant addition of the multiplied values of the different cells is termed as the Maturation Value (M.V.) It was first introduced by deLaguna (1958) and described by Frost (1958). It is as shown in the example in Table 4.1 below.

Table 4.1: Differential Count

P	I	S
0	40	60

For example

Superficial cells 60 × 1 = 60

Intermediate 40 × 0.5 = 20

Parabasal 0.0 × 0 = 0.0

After calculation, as shown below the result is MaturationValue (MV)

MV = 20 + 60 = 80

In the first half of the menstrual cycle at the peak level of oestrogen, is classically seen high (varies from 40 to 80 %), on the 15th day of the menstrual cycle.

This index shows the oestrogen effect, hence it was previously known as "Oestrogen Value." The term "Oestrogen Value" was used as a misnomer by Meisels till 1966; later, in 1967, he suggested the name Maturation Value of Frost. Meisels further stated (1968) that he found the Maturation Value as the most useful index for the purpose of coding and computing data from a large number of patients by means of an electronic ordinator. In research projects, correlations could be established and significance levels calculated for data obtained from large numbers of patients.

II. Progesterone Effect

a. If the epithelium is first primed by oestrogen and has already reached the maturation stage, that is, it contains mostly pyknotic superficial cells, the progesterone as an **antagonist** causes regression of the epithelium to the intermediate cell layer.This is observed in the second half of themenstrual cycle.

b. If fertilization occurs, then the regression continues and further proliferation stops at the Intermediate cells level on account of its dual action as antagonist and synergist, in the first trimester of pregnancy. This leads to increase in the exfoliation of the Intermediate cells in the second and third trimester.

c. Further, progesterone predominance is seen in the smear in the form of heavy exfoliation of intermediate cells along with **placard formation**.

d. In addition to heavy exfoliation, there is curling and folding of the mature squamous cells,known as the **Envelope effect**

e. Some of the intermediate cells are **modified to navicular cells**

f. **Deoderlein bacilli** appear, increase in number and cause cytolysis, leucocytes also appear and the background now becomes dirty.

g. In case pregnancy does not occur during the luteal phase of the menstrual cycle, there is hormonal withdrawal as a result of the degeneration of the corpusluteum, which leads to withdrawal bleeding (as Menstruation).

h. **Semi quantitative Assesment of the Predominance of Progesterone:** In the luteal phase of the menstrual cycle and in the different trimesters of pregnancy, it can be judged by the following indices (as shown in diagram 4.5 and 4.6)

i. CCI – Crowded Cell Index
ii. FCI – Folded Cell Index
iii. Navicular Cell Count and Index

1. **Crowded Cell Index:** This index represents the relation of the mature squamous cells, lying in clusters of four or more in comparison to clusters of three or less crowded mature cells (Table 4.1). This index is cumbersome to assess and is often similar to folded cell index.

2. **The Folded Cell Index:** This index represents the relation of all folded mature, squamous cells to flat squamous (mature) cells.

3. **Navicular Cell Count:** Papanicolaou originally described these as

navicular cell of pregnancy (1925). These are modified intermediate cells with heavy glycogen deposit in the cytoplasm. These cells have a delicate cytoplasm, thickened cell borders and small oval eccentrically placed nuclei. They exhibit a pronounced tendency to cluster formation. In the Papanicolaou stain these appear as pale blue or green; thesecells increase with the predominance of progesterone,in the luteal phase of the menstrual cycle and in pregnancy.

According to Papanicolaou there is no striking difference between the navicular cells occurring in normal pregnancy and those seen innonpregnant women inthe luteal phase of the menstrual cycle. But Wachtel and Terzano (1968) have mentioned in their observations that navicuar cells in a pregnant woman seem to be smaller and to have a much heavier looking membrane, while those found during the luteal phase of the menstrual cycle are larger and more navicular in shape. However Shamim, while working on a project on Hormonal Cytology in Pregnancy (for her MD thesis, 1974–75), found a characteristic navicular shape or typical boat shaped navicular cell (Microphotograph 4.1) in

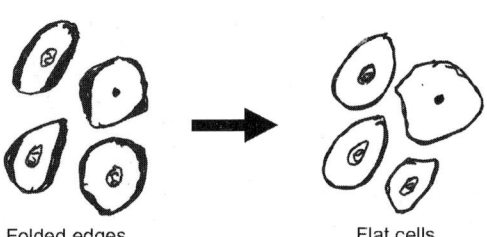

Collection of more than 3 in a group   Collection of less than 3 in one group

Diagram. 4.5: Crowded cell index (CCI)

Folded edges   Flat cells

Diagram. 4.6: Folded cell index (FCI)

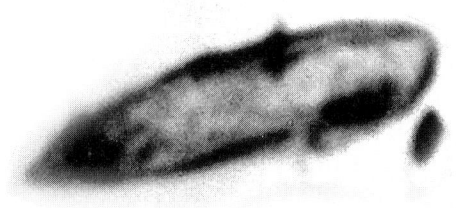

Microphotograph 4.1: Boat shaped Navicular Cell in Urinary Sediment Smear

the urine of a pregnant female.In routine work permy observations, I am in agreement with Papanicolaou, although in some cases one or two cells take the shape of typical pregnancy cells (Wachtel 1969), in addition to the groups of navicular cells as described by Papanicolaou.

Navicular Cell Index: It is the percentage of navicular cells in the smear.

Besides the above mentioned changes, in pregnancy, there is also a reduction in the KPI; in addition,the cervical mucous becomes opaque, shows the presence of numerous leucocytes and loses its elasticity. Deoderlien bacilli grow in large numbers. The smears in the luteal phase mainly consist of intermediate cells which show high glycogen content. Glycogen is the chief nutrition for the Doderlein bacilli. In order to obtain the glycogen found in the intermediate cells, the Doderlein bacilli cause cytolysis of these cells. Thus the background becomes dirty during the luteal phase.

Wied, del Sol and Dragan (1958) suggested that FCI and CCI may be used as additional records in assessing cell criteria, while Meisels (1967) stated that Frost's Maturation Index when combined with CCI and FCI during the luteal phase will be most helpful in diagnosis, since it will reflect the changes of the epithelium under multi hormonal effect.

Androgen: This is a male hormone, which is usually synthesized in the ovary in very small amounts by the modified theca interna. These cells then transfer the androgen to the granulosa cells which convert it to oestrogen. Physiologically, androgen is produced in small amounts directly by the adrenal cortex throughout the reproductive period of life. It is found in such miniscule doses during the reproductive period that the hormone does not produce any effect on the normal vaginal smear pattern.

After menopause, androgen is secreted in high doses. Its effect on vaginal smears is similar to high doses of progesterone,showing intermediate cell proliferation, but it is without the curling, folding and crowding effect. This effect may be observed in young castrated women, who in the immediate post-operative period showatrophy of vaginal smear cells, but later show a spontaneous return to the proliferative phase with low KPI. This is because the metabolite of androgen behaves like oestrogen, except that it produces a predominance of intermediate cells. Frequently androgenic type cells (Gompel and Pundal, 1957) appear in the vaginal smear, which is due to compensatory hormonal secretion of androgen.

The androgenic type of cell is a cyanophilic intermediate cell with pale cytoplasm, often vacuolated and with a large regular hypochromatic nucleus. Normally in these cases the absence of eosinophilicpyknotic cells and leucocytes is quite characteristic (Pundal 1957). I have observed during routine hormonal evaluation that the presence of an isolated Androgen cell (Microphotograph 4.2) in a normally progressing pregnancy, was seen earliest at 7 weeks. It was possibly significant in those cases, where the pregnant woman was carrying a female foetus (Khan, Ahmad and Rizvi 1975).

Clinically, cytology is helpful in establishing the effective dose of androgen as therapy. The dose is established when the

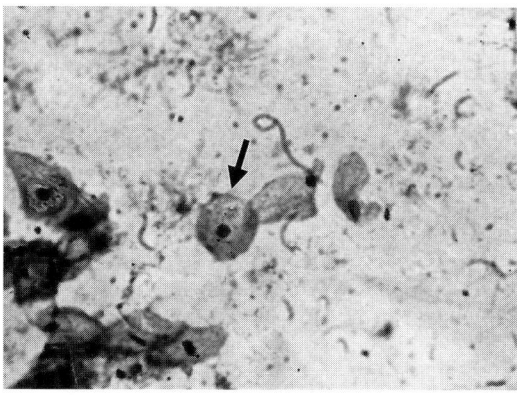

Microphotograph No 4.2: Androgen cell (at arrow) at seven weeks of pregnancy

hormone changes the atrophic smear to the proliferation of the intermediate cell. The speed with which the changes occur and the persistence of pattern depends on the various types of androgenic hormone.

Other Steroid Hormones: Pituitary gonadotrophic hormones have no direct effect on the vaginal smear. These primarily act on the ovary through the FSH and LH hormones. The ovary responds to the FSH and LH hormones by secreting oestrogen and progesterone. In case of failure of the pituitary gland, FSH and LH are not produced. Pergonal is given exogenously and if ovaries are functioning, a proliferative effect is seen. Later the administration of LH promotes the formation of corpus luteum, which secretes the progesterone, causing proliferative effect. This can be observed in the vaginal smears.

Cortisone and ACTH have no influence on the vaginal epithelium.

Chorionic Gonadotrophins: These are secreted by the placental trophoblastic cells. Their action alone and directly on the vaginal epithelium is not known. In pregnancy, these hormones produce an effect on the vaginal smear cells probably, through progesterone.

The effect of all these hormones on the vulva and the urinary bladder epithelia is identical to the effect on the vaginal epithelium, as these three epithelia embryologically originate from the same source that is from the urogenital sinus. The vulval smear shows a high KPI while the urinary sediment smear though scanty, shows negligible infection in comparison to the higher infection seen in the vaginal cells.

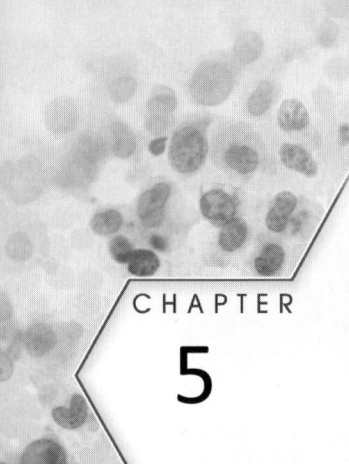

Evaluation of Indices Used for the Assessment of Oestrogen and Progesterone Effect

I. Oestrogen

1. Karyopyknotic Index: This represents the percentage of superficial cells with pyknotic nucleus (5 – 6µ)among 200 – 400 unselected squamous cells, excluding the parabasal cell sunder the magnification x 40 objective. This index is utilized to observe the response of the vaginal epithelium to stimulation by oestrogen. This index is constant and highly specific so that it can be used for the hormonal assessment of the first half of the normal menstrual cycle, and its disorders as well as normal pregnancy and its disorders, for example, abortion. This test can also be utilized for assessing the therapeutic potency of unknown oestrogens.

All other methods (other indices) of expressing the oestrogenic effect are also based on the maturing effect, that is, the Maturation index and the Maturation value.

Maturation Index: It represents the differential cell count of squamous cell population and is expressed as a percentage. Counts of at least 200 (or 400) cells are made in the representative fields, using x40 objective, including the parabasal, intermediate and superficial cells per 100 cells and is recorded in the following manner (Table 5.2).

Table 5.2		
Shift to Left Mostly Immature	← (P) (I) (S)	Shift to Right – Mostly Mature Cells

Erica Wachtel (1969) mentioned that a single observation of an index alone or in different combinations of indices are not of much value in infertility, amenorrhoea, premenopausal period or even in pregnancy, when under the effect of multiple hormones. Therefore it is advised to obtain serial smears in such cases to understand the underlying disease process.

Ruiz (1968) also gave his opinion during a discussion at the symposium on hormonal cytology (1968) that the study of an isolated index in one smear (as usually requested by the physician) is of little diagnostic value, rathera serial smear study for 3 – 4 menstrual cycles in amenorrhoea and 3 – 4 weeks in menopausal patients is essential.

In specific conditions even a single index, such as KPI serial smears provides useful and reliable information of oestrogen effect when there is no interference from the other sex hormones, that is, progesterone, androgen or chorionic gonadotrophins.

The conditions under which the assessment of a single index provides valuable information are:

1. For demonstration of ovulation in the first half of the menstrual cycle (Pre and post-ovulatory checkup).
2. To differentiate between the types of anovulatory cycles in infertility and amenorrhoea.

3. Before Menarche and in childhood to recognize abnormal oestrogen effect.

4. In menopause for purposes of classification and to understand the underlying hormonal interplay.

5. In cases of suspected feminizing tumour – as an aid in the diagnosis.

6. For follow up in patients subsequent to treatment for oestrogen producing tumour. In these cases, the index serves as a reliable indicator for recurrence.

7. The KPI is helpful in therapy monitoring and prognosis in the following cases.
   a. Assessment of the success of androgen therapy in Breast Cancer.
   b. Radiation treatment of malignant diseases of the female genital tract.
   c. In patients undergoing treatment for threatened abortion, amenorrhoea and menopause.
   d. In Turner's syndrome to avoid over dosage of hormone therapy.Since over dosage leads to premature epiphyseal fusion and arrests growth of child in Turner's syndrome.
   e. In breast cancer, the KPI indicates the requirement of androgen in order to achieve hormonal castration in patients.

Limitation in the study of Hormonal assessment by the vaginal cytology study are as follows:

1. Vaginal infection which is common in Multiparous patients, particularly TV infestations, cause excessive maturing effect. The degenerating effect of the infection on superficial cells causes increased pyknotic effect, while the hyperaemia associated with infection, causes rapid maturation of the superficial cells.

2. Digitalis therapy has a maturing effect. The action is through its active principle factor, the chemical structure of which resembles oestrogen.

3. In cases where abstinence is not observed for 48 hours prior to the test, the results may not be reliable.

4. If douches and pessaries are used within 24 hours of the test, the results again are unreliable.

5. In patients of liver disease, oestrogen is not eliminated from the circulation, these high levels of circulating hormones lead to excessive maturation.

6. In cases where prolonged treatment with high doses of oestrogen is given, the KPI reverses to low levels.

II. Progesterone

Rubenstein (1940) Neustaedter (1940) and Brown (1949) and Pundal (1959) and many other workers found that vaginal smear changes are an approximate gauge of oestrogen activity, while application of the same techniques could not find unanimous favour in the determination of progesterone activity. We also observed that vaginal epithelium response to progesterone is inconsistent, hence it is an unreliable assessment tool.

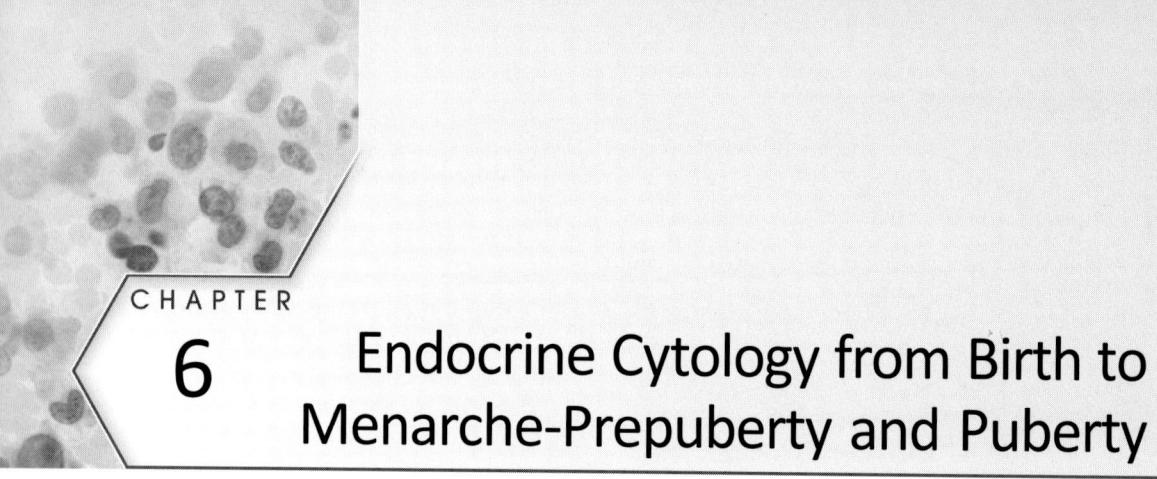

Endocrine Cytology from Birth to Menarche-Prepuberty and Puberty

Endocrine cytology reflects the diverse hormonal profile of a female during the different phases of life from birth to Menopause.

The vaginal epithelium changes serially throughout the life of a female subject as shown by Miniello and Saraiya in their Atlas of Cytology and Colposcopy (1998) in Diagram 6.1 (Fig. 4.8 of Atlas). These physiological changes are in response to the changing hormone production at different phases (abcde) of life.

The endocrine cytology from Birth to Menopause can be discussed in the following three groups:

1. **Birth to Menarche (i to vi)**

2. **Reproductive Period** (a) Menstrual cycle –Ovulatory and Anovulatory (b) Pregnancy and its disorders.

3. **Menopause:** (includes Pre, and Post menopausal phases.)

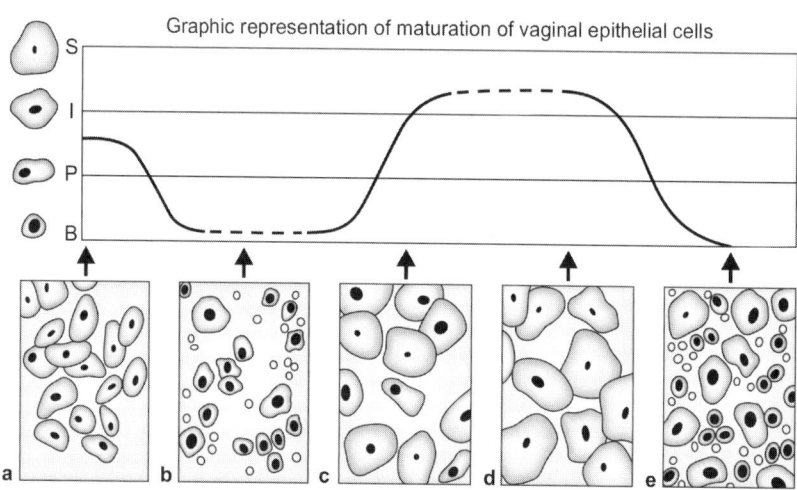

Diagram 6.1: Vaginal cells palterns in different stages of life (Upper part) shows the graphic representation of maturation of vaginal epithelium (lower part a,b,c,d,e.) shows the vaginal cells pattern in different phases of life: (a) Epithelial Maturation at birth; (b) Atrophic pattern in childhood; (c) Beginning of oestrogenic influence in puberty; (d) Complete maturation in the reproductive period; (e) Regression in old age.

I. ENDOCRINE CYTOLOGY FROM "BIRTH TO MENARCHE

i. At birth

a. Vaginal smear shows copious exfoliation of intermediate cells;

b. There are a fair number of superficial cells under the effect of the mother's oestrogen, present in the blood of the newborn;

c. Karyopyknotic index – up to 20% (Wachtel and Plester 1952) with a clean background due to the absence of leucocytes, mucin and Deoderlein bacilli.

ii. 2nd to 4th day after birth

A mixed picture of Intermediate Cells and parabasalcellswith moderate cytolysis of cells, and bacteria as well as leucocytes are now seen in the vaginal smears (Wachtel 1969).

Dr Saraiya in a panel discussion of IAC (1969), described the normal hormonal changes in a female child from birth to menarche and divided these changes into 4 classical phases:

First Phase – Hyperhormonal post natal phase, which is to from **birth to the 5th day**. She observed in it, a high KPI and abundant Intermediate cells, as reported by Wachtel and Plester (1952). The reason explained by Dr Saraiya, was same as found by the others, that high concentration of maternal oestrogen transmitted across the placental membranes during the foetal life, was still circulating in the blood of the newborn.

iii. 5th to 7th day after birth

a. Intermediate cells decrease or disappear from the vaginal smears.

b. A few RBCs are seen (Boschann - 1960) due to withdrawal of mother's oestrogen from the circulation of the newborn.

c. Bacteria and Leucocytes steadily increase in number in the vaginal smears, (Wachtel 1969)

iv. 7th to 8th day

a. Atrophic vaginal smear (Parabasal cells only)

b. Complete elimination of Hormones, resulting in a rapid fall in KPI by day 8 (as shown in diagram 6.2) (Wachtel 1969).

Dr Saraiya has labelled the period from 5th to 8th day as the Second phase of massive vaginal regression or genital crisis. In this phase, Dr Saraiya found that bacterial invasion takes place and the background now is dirty; the Superficial cells disappear, the placard becomes smaller and there is abundant massive desquamation of cells. Certain amount of hemorrhage may occur, which is certainly the result of sudden withdrawal of maternal oestrogen.

v. 9 to 15th day

In vaginal smears, a complete atrophy persists showing parabasal cell, a pattern which is maintained throughout infancy and childhood (approximately the age of 9 years).

Dr Saraiya has split up the period from the 8th day to the age of Puberty into two phases:

Dr Saraiya has labelled the period from the 8th to the 15th day as the Third phase of Installation of Prepubertal phase, in which Parabasal cells make their appearance and Deoderlein bacilli are well established. The Intermediate cells start decreasing.

According to Dr Saraiya, the Fourth phase is the Prepubertal phase, which starts from the 2nd week onwards after birth. In this phase, the atrophic pattern of the Prepubertal phase will typify the vaginal smear during

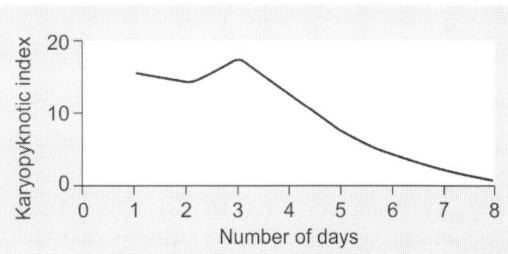

Diagram 6.2: Shows colpocytogram of a new born up to the day 8 (Wachtel 1969)

childhood, when the slow regeneration and the lack of protective action by the large squamous cells along with the absence of lactobacillus, makes the vaginal mucosa, fragile and liable to infections. This smear pattern continues till puberty, when endogenous oestrogen production starts.

vi. Pre-Puberty and Puberty (9–15 years)

Vaginal hormonal cytology study in these phaseshas been given very little attention in English medical literature. **Sonek (1967)** was the first one to study the prepubertal as well as pubertal vaginal cytology. He found only one detailed study of the cytodiagnosis of the female child in a paper (in French language) by DeBrux and Delsace (1958), after search of world literature.

Sonek in 1967 has extensively studied the Prepuberty period from 9 to 12 years and described it in great detail; in addition, he has described a special technique for the collection of smears from the fragile vagina of childhood as shown in Diagram 6.3.

A glass pipette was used, through which a small cotton applicator was introduced into the vagina, so that it did not make contact with the vulva or the ectocervix and directly reached the lateral vaginal wall. Speculum should not be employed in children.

In routine practice, the cotton applicator can be used directly to prepare a smear without the glass pipette but an experienced cytopathologist is required to differentiate the contamination caused through the ectocervix and the vulva and discard it from the results of the hormonal assessment. Further the difference between the proliferative states of the epithelia found in the upper part of vagina when compared to the lower portion, does not play a significant role in the assessment of the cytologic pattern in smears from children. These smears are fixed in isopropyl alcohol and stained by Shorrs (1941). Evaluation of the smears is carried out by the method of Schmitt (1953) with some modifications.

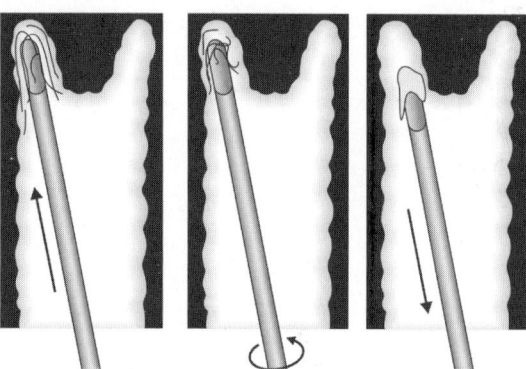

Preparation technique of specimen in female children (Sonek 1967)

Diagram 6.3: Technique of collection of specimen

Prepubertal Phase: (age 9–12 years)

The period three to four years prior to the onset of Menstruation at Menarche is known as the Pre-Pubertal period.

The vaginal smear patterns studied by Sonek (1967) showed that the increase in the proliferation of cells was not continuously progressive, hence most smears were of mixed cell type. Further, there was irregularity of cellular proliferation, as characterized by the variation of cell size among the same type of cells. Superficial cells were sometimes found as giant cells with binucleation. During this period, the duration of the menstrual cycle were either prolonged or decreased. and were not regular as that observed in the normal cycle. Very few cases of stabilized cyclic changes were found in female children between 9 and 12 years.

Puberty: (age 12–15 years) The pattern studied by Sonek (1967) from serial vaginal smears in puberty was as follows:

A. Ovulatory cycles – A few cases (5.9%)

B. Anovulatory cycles – 90.6% (rest Indistinct)

The hormonal cytology of the girls with anovulatory cycle was of the following types:

1. Normo – oestrogenic* 44.1%

2. Hypo – oestrogenic 20.8%

3. Hyper – oestrogenic** 31.2%

4. Irregular 3.9%

*Majority of the cases were of Normo – oestrogenic type followed by the Hyper-oestrogenic type, while the Hypo-oestrogenic type was the least of all cases.

The epithelial cycle during puberty is usually characterized by great variability and lability. Lability is the consequence of the various disturbances of the menstrual cycle, which require to be assessed at this age with great care and treated with conservative methods.

It is to be noted that a hyper-oestrogenic** oligomenorrhea may progress to an amenorrhoeic condition, which in turn may proceed to a hyper-oestrogenic metrorrhagia. In serial examinations, the hyper-oestrogenic disturbances of the cycle exhibit a typical pattern labelled as cytologic hyper-oestrogenic syndrome of a juvenile female.

1. During amenorrhoeic phase.

a. Isolation and maximal enlargement of cells leads to increase in number to such an extent that cells lie side by side, mostly without folding. There is cytoplasmic granulation and for-mation of a perinuclear halo, which indicates the persistent oestrogen effect.

Later there is a loss of cellular turgor which results in:

1. a. Irregular shapes V or Y or infolding of cellular margins. These in turn suggest a decrease in oestrogenic effect.

b. Withdrawal of hormone results in:

i. Bleeding Per Vaginum, that is, withdrawal bleeding

ii. The KPI - falls

11. More marked changes are often observed in the cells, as follows:

a. Increase alteration of cytoplasmic configuration

b. Further reduction in cellular turgor, which sometimes causes degeneration.

c. Development of fine fissions in cytoplasm or marked folding resembling pleats.

Among the individual disturbances of the cycle during puberty, besides oligomenorrhea, secondary amenorrhoea may occur with hypo-oestrogenic cycles, either slight or moderate, which require occasional proper examination. Of the remaining cyclic dysfunction, only markedly hypoestrogenic cases require special attention, if this occurs at the age of 15 yrs.

During Puberty special attention is given to certain cytologic criteria, which occur fairly frequently.

1. Rod like nuclei (Sonek 1967)

2. Leaf like phenomenon (Hopman 1959), which has been observed also in Pregnancy ; or

3. Spoon like phenomenon (Papanicolaou 1941) described in pregnancy.

4. The other changes are as follows.

• The vesicular nucleus exhibits a flattened outline so that it assumes an oval shape.

• The chromatin structure is dense along the major axis of oval shaped nucleus, forming a central line.

• During the further stages of nuclear degeneration, one observes small processes, deriving from the central line.

• With further flattening of the nucleus and increased density of the chromatin structure, the nucleus become elongated, dark and rod shaped. The consistency is sometimes opaque as found in Karyopyknotic nucleus.

Vaginal cytology is simple, painless, and serial examination is easily performed; thus it has been found to be an especially useful gynecological assessment tool during puberty and prepubertal phases in female children.

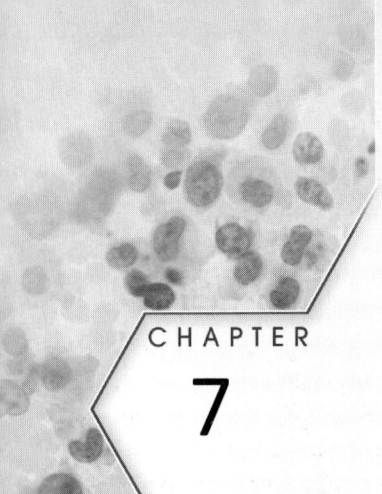

Endocrine Cytology During the Reproductive Period

MENSTRUAL CYCLE

The Vaginal smear pattern changes due to cyclical variation of the ovarian hormones during the menstrual cycle; thus it indirectly informs the functional state of the ovary.

The Menstrual cycle can be both (a) Ovulatory (b) Anovulatory.

1. Ovulation Pattern

There is the proliferative phase during which, under the effect of FSH, there is oestrogen production alone (refer to Hypothalamus-Pituitary–Ovarian axis chapter).. When the production of oestrogen is at the peak on the 14th day (classical day) of the cycle (ovulation period varies from the 12 – 19th day of the Menstrual Cycle), and the KPI is maximum (60 to 80%), ovulation occurs. According to Wachtel and Plester (1952) KPI rarely exceeds 40 %, while De Allende and Orias (1950) and Pundal (1952) have reported a KPI of 80 – 90 %at the time of ovulation. In our series, we have found a KPI of 40–60% on an average in most cases.

Proliferative phase of the vaginal smear shows:

a. Predominance of discretely arranged superficial polyhedral cells
b. The cytoplasm of these cells is clear and transparent

c. The cells have well defined borders with eosinophilic cytoplasm and pyknotic nuclei
d. The background is clean, without leucocytes or bacteria
e. Intermediate and pre-cornified cells are few in number
f. There is no clustering of cells and in cases where the superficial cells over lap, the borders of the underlying cells are visible through the transparent cytoplasm of the cells above them

This is the phase of unopposed oestrogen activity.

The features of the proliferative phase can be seen in anovulatory cycles under the following conditions:

a. Persistent follicular cyst
b. Hyperoestrogenwhich is associated with endometrial hyperplasia
c. Oestrogen producing tumours
d. Following administration of exogenous Oestrogen

Secretory Phase

In the postovulatory phase, the corpora haemorrhagica of the ovary is transformed into a Corpus Luteum, under the effect of Luteinizing Hormone (LH). Progesterone is now secreted in large amounts with little oestrogen secretion and this changes the proliferative phase to a secretory phase.

Under the predominant effect of progesterone, there is reversion of the superficial squamous epithelial cells to intermediate cells, without further development and maturity of these cells. This phase is characterized by an excessive proliferation of the intermediate cells.

The Smears Show:

1. Heavy exfoliation of the intermediate cells (Cyanophilic).
2. The intermediate cells contains a large amount of glycogen, deposited in their cytoplasm.
3. On account of the glycogen deposition in the intermediate cells, the cytoplasm becomes transparent and the nucleus gets pushed to the periphery.
4. 10 – 15 percent of the intermediate cells transform into Navicular cells.
5. The Navicular cells found during the menstrual cycle are larger and more navicular in shape while those found during pregnancy, are smaller and have thickened cell borders (Terzano–1968).
6. The KPI drops down 15-30%.
7. EI is also low at 10 – 15%.
8. There is cluster formation of intermediate cells.
9. There is marked curling and folding of cell edges called the Envelope effect
10. On account of deposition of glycogen in the cells, there is heavy growth of the Deoderlein bacilli.
11. Heavy growth of Deoderlein bacilli causes cytolysis. Hence naked nuclei are seen.
12. The background is dirty, due to conversion of elastic mucous into a tacky opaque secretion, rich in leucocytes and the naked cell nuclei
13. CCI and FCI increase.
14. Maturation index–this shows a shift to mid zone, in the secretory phase of the menstrual cycle (Table 7.1).

Table 7.1: Shift towards the intermediate cells

0	91	10
00	85	15

Menstrual Phase: When the progestational phase reaches the 28th day of the cycle, the corpus luteum degenerates and hormone withdrawal leads to menstruation.

The menstrual smear is characterized by:

a. Endometrial cells admixed with blood
b. Intermediate cells, which in the beginning show clustering, folding and crowding, thereafter disappear
c. Maximum shedding occurs on the second/third day of the menstrual cycle
d. There is heavy exfoliation of the endometrial cells and these are seen in the blood after the second/third day of the menstrual cycle
e. There is occasional cell degeneration leading to cytoplasmic vacuolation
f. At the end of menstruation, histocy tesappear, which later become numerous. These engulf debris, erythrocytes and blood pigments

The postmenstrual phase again shows a gradual effect of oestrogen activity and the cycle starts, repeating the proliferation followed by the secretory phase and the menstrual phase.

These cycles are repeated again and again till pregnancy occurs or if not, till menopause sets in.

Normal Ovulatory Menstrual Cycle

The Karyopyknotic index curves were obtained by plotting the KPI against the days of the menstrual cycle as shown in (diagrams 7.1 A and B. (Wachtel 1969).

For the confirmation of Ovulation: Intracytoplasmic lipid granules were observed in the

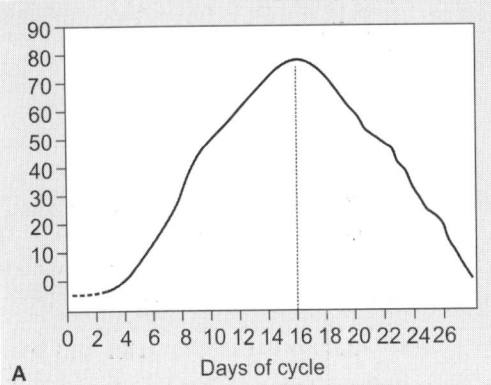

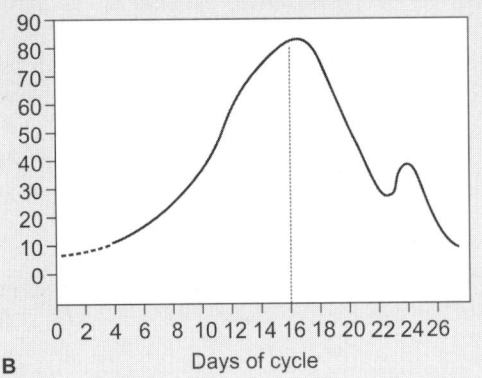

Diagrams 7.1A and B: Normal Ovulatory Cycle patterns these curves show a progressive rise to peak value followed by a sharp decrease which is as represented in (A) or may show secondary rise of short deviation as seen in (B)

vaginal cells by Malliet et al in 1978. These were found to be a sensitive indicator of the post ovulatory phase. He carried out a clinical study of 190 women (1978) and found that intracytoplasmic lipid granules, stained with oil Red revealed a different profile under the effect of oestrogen and progesterone. These findings are in agreement with the study of Ebne et al 1954, Masin et al 1964, and Tapazov (1965).

Cyclic variation of intracytoplasmic lipid granules in the phases of menstrual cycle and in different conditions is shown below in table 7.2.

II. The profile of Intracytoplasmic granules in other conditions is as follows:

1. Women taking oral contraceptive
2. Stein Leventhal syndrome
3. In pregnancy
4. In post menopausal women
5. Anovulatorymenstrual cycle
6. In Late Menopause

Lipid granules are scarce (+) in 90 – 100% cells, smaller than 1µ showed irregular distribution without clustering

Menstrual cycles	Intracytoplasmic lipid granules in normal ovulatory cycles				
	Percentage of granules in the cells	Number of granules in each cell	Diameter of each Granule	Distribution of granules in cells	Confluence/ Clustering of granules
First half of menstrual cycle – 1st – 15th day	100%	+ +	Smaller then 1u	Regular	Absent
2nd half of menstrual cycle 20 – 25th day	100%	+ + +	Larger than 1u	Irregular	Present

Table 7.2: Cyclic Variation of Intracytoplasmic Lipid Granules

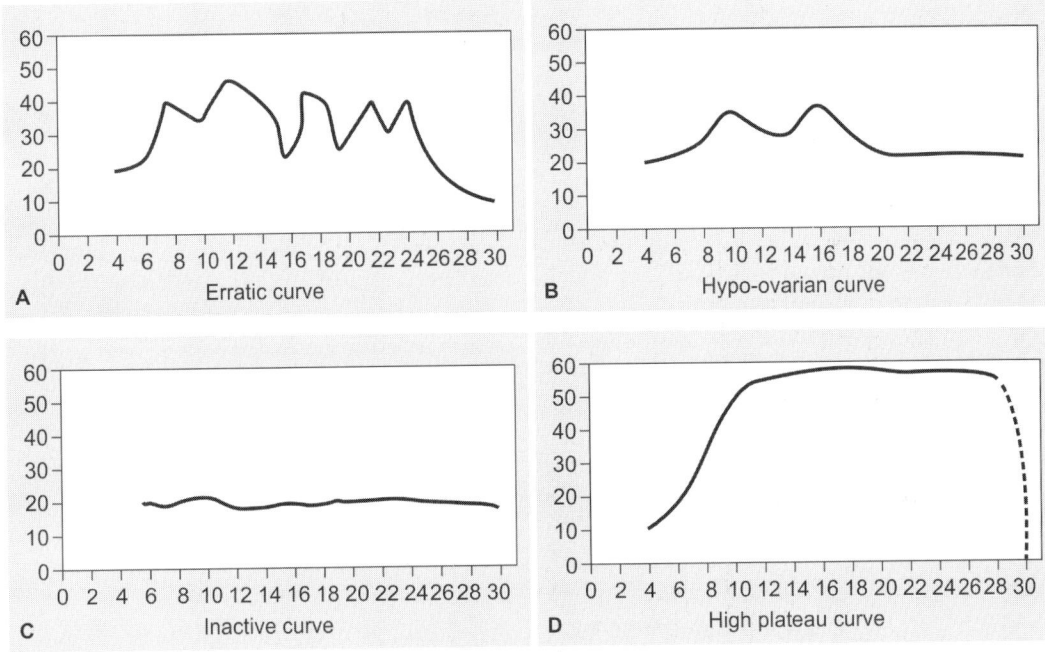

Diagram 7.2A to D

2. Anovulatory Menstrual Cycle

Anovulatory curves are observed when the proliferative phase is not followed by the secretory phase since ovulation does not occur. However, the withdrawal of oestrogen leads to withdrawal bleeding. Anovulatory curves show great individual variation, reflecting the degree of ovarian disturbance, thus permitting speculation on the prognosis of the disorder. Four types of anovulatory curves are recognized (Wachtel, 1969) as shown in Diagram 7.2 A to D .

1. **Erratic Curve** is characterized by irregular fluctuations indicating variation in oestrogen secretion. These can be observed as occasional anovulatory cycles in an otherwise normally ovulating woman who is approaching menopause. It is rarely a frequent finding in premenopausal women (Diagram 7.2A)

2. **Hypo-Ovarian Curve:** It is characterized by low karyopyknotic index (KPI) values, which indicate severe ovarian disturbance (Diagram 7.2B).

3. **The Inactive Curve:** It is characterized by flatness with a complete absence of fluctuations and low karyopyknotic index readings. This type of curve is found in patients whose ovaries are not functioning and is identical with those from post menopausal women (Diagram. 7.2C)

4. **High Plateau Curve:** It is defined as a curve without significant fluctuations but with high readings of KPI. There is often a normal progressive rise at the start until a peak value is reached which value is maintained for a considerable period of time. A sudden steep drop in the curve is followed by bleeding (withdrawal bleeding–not menstruation). Such curves are common in the presence of persistent follicular cyst and oestrogen producing tumours (Diagram 7.2D).

These anovulatory cycles are also important from the point of view of infertility.

The relation of vaginal cytology to the varying hormonal functions have been studied by several investigators. Most of these workers agree upon the well defined response to oestrogen. In the management of infertility in a female, it is of fundamental importance to distinguish whether one is dealing with a case of ovulatory failure or whether one has to look elsewhere for the cause of infertility. The classical premenstrual endometrial biopsy is evidence of secretory activity which is diagnostic of successful ovulation. However it was found to be a painful, traumatic, costly and time consuming surgical procedure. Further it had to be performed by an experienced gynecologist in a hospital setting. On the other hand, exfoliative cytology study of the vaginal, vulvalor and urinary sediment smear are an easy, speedy, nontraumic and economic procedures. In anovulatory cycles (as shown in Diagram 7.2A to D) the follicle having reached a particular stage of its development begins to regress without having ruptured. Thus ovulation does not occur. Now this can also be confirmed by the post ovulatory intra cytoplasm lipid granule test (Malliet et al 1978). The menstrual flow in such cases is of the nature of an oestrogen withdrawal bleeding, as the corpus luteum is not formed and there is no progesterone secretion.

Garud and Saraiya et al carried out cytohormonal evaluation of 100 infertility cases with anovulatroy cycles in 1978 and later Saraiya et al further studied the serial vaginal-cytology in 130 infertile women with ovulatory cycles in 1979. In both these groups, vaginal cytology and cervical mucus viscosity and elasticity were studied to find out the exact day of ovulation, which they found varied from 10 to 19 days in different patients. Although the study of cervical mucus for the evidence of ovulation was found to be a useful tool but on comparision of merits and demerits of both the methods they felt that cytology was more helpful.

In the anovulatory group serial cytological studies help them in deciding the degree of ovarian failure. Cases with hyper oestrogenic and normo oestrogenic smears were selected for Clomiphene Citrate therapy. 8 out of 100 cases (anovulatory group) became pregnant. They found that in the absence of basal temperature charts, KPI as judged by vaginal cytology and cervical mucus studies help them to select the patients for Clomiphene Citrate therapy.

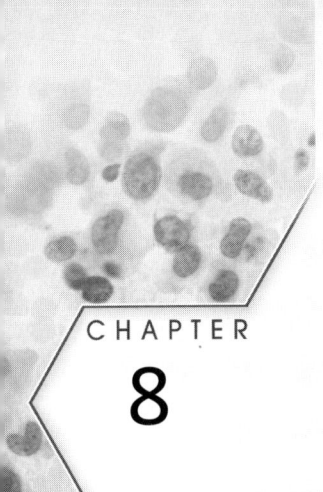

Endocrine Cytology of Normal Pregnancy

Normal Pregnancy: Papanicolaou (1925) was the first person to publish vaginal smear data on the hormonal changes in a pregnant female. Since then, vaginal cytology has been ascribed great importance as the vaginal epithelium was found to be the most sensitive indicator of hormonal changes in pregnancy. Further it was established as a reliable method by several workers, including Pundal (1959), Spira and Mac Rae (1960), Wood, Osmond – Clarke and Murray (1961), VonHaam (1961), Soule (1964), Meisels (1966), and Teter and Teter (1968). Wachtel (1969) in her book stated that endocrine cytology is a rewarding technique, when applied throughout the gestational period.

Papanicolaou (1948) noticed the cytological uniformity between the vaginal and urinary sediment smears. Many workers, Sora (1959), Lencioni (1963, 1969), O. Morchoe and O Morchoe (1967), Pinto et al. (1968), Mitra et al. (1974), (1975) noted comparable findings in hormonal cytology of these two techniques during pregnancy. They considered the urinary cytology as an advancement over the vaginal cytology method. Later Delcastillo and Videla (1966) described the process of cellular desquamation from the inner surface of the labia minora (Nymphae), similar to that demonstrated through urinary and vaginal cytology. Reports on vulval cytology (Nymphocytogram) are few, as reported by

Dennerstein (1968), Pinto et al (1968), Videla (1969) and Tozzini et al (1971).

Pinto et al were the first to study the Nymphocytogram in pregnancy. They also carried out a comparative study of vaginal, vulval and urinary sediment smears in pregnancy utilizing only EI and KPI for statistical comparison (1968). Later (1977), Shamim, Khan, and Rizvi reported a study of hormonocytology of pregnancy with a comparative statistical evaluation of the colpocytogram, nymphocytogram and urocytogram utilizing KPI, MV, CCI and FCI (graphs, as shown in diagram 8.1 and 8.2. In these graphs nymphocytogram, as well as the urinary sediment smears show identical results when compared with colpocytogram, except that there are high KPI and MV values at the beginning of first trimester of pregnancy in the nymphocytogram. This may be attributable to the fact that the vulval epithelium is more mature, and hence less sensitive to the low hormonal levels of early pregnancy (Dennerstein, 1968).

Inspite of the fact that all three techniques showed identical results and follow the same pattern in all three trimesters, the urinary sediment smear on observation appeared a more accurate method of determining the hormonal activity. Urinary sediment smear could easily replace colpocytograms in cases of vaginal bleeding and infection. Thus is due

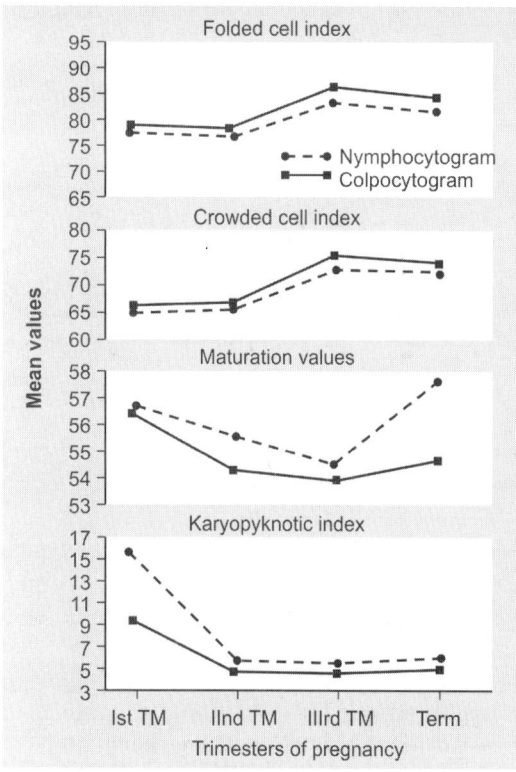

Comparative statistical study of cellular curves
in different trimester of pregnancy

Diagram 8.1:

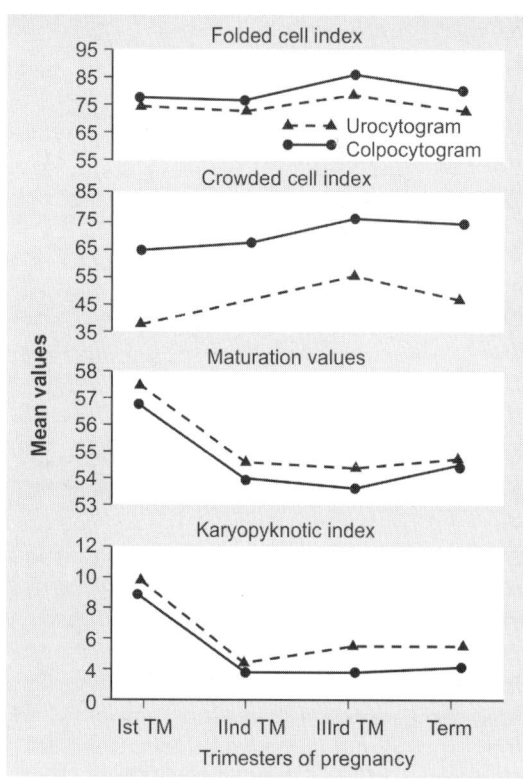

Comparative statistical study of cellular curves
in different trimester of pregnancy

Diagram 8.2:

to the fact that the urinary sediment smears, especially the catheter specimen, are free from infection and blood which is a definite advantage over the colpocytogram. Although there is a low sensitivity of the urinary epithelium to hormones, the significant cytologic changes in hormonal levels can be easily noted. The recognition and identi-fication of cells is indeed easier and less equivocal in the urinary sediment smears. Thus it could easily replace colpocytogram, whenever required.

MacRae (1967) tried to correlate vaginal cytology with urinary hormone assay in normal as well as in abnormal cases of pregnancy. He concluded that that the response of the cells was a more authentic guide to hormone action rather than the estimation of hormone excretion. It has been noted that whenever there is poor response to hormone treatment, enzyme block may be suspected (experimental work of Talwar and Saigal 1963).

Although Wachtel (1968) reported that in rare circumstances, pregnancy smears may show grossly abnormal cytology, that is, high KPI, intermediate cells without curling and folding and the absence of navicular cells. Perhaps the vaginal epithelium in these cases is refractory to hormonal stimuli or it may be the consequence of an enzyme block, as mentioned earlier.

Hormonal Changes in Pregnancy: At the discussion of the Hypothalamus – Pituitary – Ovarian axis, it was explained that in the post fertilization phase, the corpus luteum persists as a temporary endocrine gland during the first trimester of pregnancy. It provides additional oestrogen and progesterone required for the maintenance of the fertilized ovum. Approximately 6 days after fertilization, implantation of the fertilized ova is complete and the developing syncytio-trophoblast of the placenta in the uterus complement the ovarian production of oestrogen and progesterone. Along with these steroids, the trophoblast commences production of chorionic gonadotrophins in the first month of pregnancy (Zender, 1959). Thus it may be assumed that the pregnancy preserving function of the corpus luteum beyond the first month of pregnancy has been overestimated.

Von Haam (1961) has mentioned that experimentally the progesterone difference between the arterial and venous placental blood in the different trimesters of pregnancy was measured via isotopic progesterone markers. In his series he has reported a progesterone production per day of 25 to 50 milligrams during the first half of pregnancy and up to 280 milligrams during the second half. The excretion of oestrogen during pregnancy also increases about 100 times as compared to that seen in the normal cycle. Brown (1956) found that the oestrogens produced by the placenta increased from 1 milligram per day in the tenth week of pregnancy to 50 to 100 milligrams per day at the end of pregnancy.

The classification of the vaginal cytology of pregnancy as proposed by Pundal (1958) was accepted by most workers in this field.

Hormono-Cytology of Pregnancy was classified into:

1. Acytolytic
2. Cytolytic

Acytolytic Pregnancy Smear Pattern

1. Cytology of the first trimester of pregnancy (upto 3 months or 12 weeks) is labeled as corpus luteum phase.
2. Cytology of the last two trimesters of pregnancy is labeled as placental phase.
   a. Placental phase extends from 12 weeks up to the last two weeks before term. This is also labelled as Preterm phase, that is up to 38 weeks of pregnancy.
   b. Cytology of pregnancy in the last 2 weeks (38 to 40 weeks) is labelled as "at term" phase (38–40 weeks).
      Kamnitzer et al (1959) opined that the classification could be expanded to comprise the entire vaginal "gravido – puerperal" cycle. Therefore they suggested the addition of one more phase after "at term" (c)
   c. Cytology at the beginning of Labour or near Term

Corpus Luteum phase—the first 12 weeks of gestation

The corpus luteum phase of the menstrual cycle after conception in the last 2 weeks of the last menstrual cycle continues as the corpus luteum phase of pregnancy, which persist until 12 week of gestation. The trophoblast of the developing placenta also aids gestation by enhancing progesterone production, from the first month onwards. The predominant hormone of pregnancy is progesterone which on account of its dual action, synergistic as well as antagonistic, allows the proliferation up to the intermediate layer and reverses the mature squamous epithelium to the intermediate cell layer, respectively. The excessive proliferation of intermediate layer leads to the following characteristic changes in the smear pattern in this phase.

Hormonal Cytology Pattern in the first trimester of pregnancy: Microphotograph 3

1. Heavy exfoliation of the intermediate cells with placard formation
2. Intermediate cells are cyanophilic, shining large flat polygonal cells with smooth

rounded edges and homogenous transparent cytoplasm. Their borders are not clearly discernable since progesterone causes agglutination of cells. The nucleus is centrally placed and oval or round. Transparency of cytoplasm is reduced because of glycogen deposition

3. **KPI:** The Karyopyknotive index drops down gradually to 10 – 15% (from 25 – 30% at the beginning of pregnancy), occasionally it may show a transient rise to 25 – 30%, which persistsfor a very short duration and then rises at monthly intervals, reflecting the persistence of cyclic activity of the ovary up to the first three months of pregnancy

4. **EI:** The Eosinophilic Index is also reduced to 5 – 10%

5. **MI:** The Maturation Index, in which the differential count shows a shift towards the mid zone in pregnancy (Table 8.1).

Table 8.1

P	I	s
0	80	20

6. **C.C.I (Crowded Cell Index):** The intermediate cells of pregnancy have tendency to crowding (grouping). Therefore CCI is defined as the "Relation of four or more cells to cells three or less in a group"

7. **F.C.I (Folded Cell Index):** The intermediate cells show curling and folding of their edges. This tendency is called the "Envelope effect. "This is enhanced and prominent

8. The background may show cytolysis and mild growth of Deoderlein bacilli

9. **Navicular Cells:** The navicular cells of the luteal phase are the modified intermediate cells. According to Pundal (1959), it would be exceptional to find the pregnancy navicular cells before the second week, following the last menstruation. These navicular cells increase 25–30% by the 12th week of pregnancy

Navicular cells are the specially modified forms of intermediate squamous cells, characterized by an oval shape and are deeply coloured towards the periphery while appearing clearer in the middle with the eccentrically placed oval or round nuclei (Ruiz 1968). The cell spossess a pronounced tendency to cluster formation (Wachtel 1968). Pundal explained that the cells are replete with glycogen which displaces the cytoplasm towards the periphery.

Pundal (1968) and Wachtel (1969) emphasized that the navicular cells are found in pregnant as well as non-pregnant females in the luteal phase of the menstrual cycle, therefore their presence in early pregnancy is not diagnostic unless confirmed by a biological or serological pregnancy test. Besides the luteal phase, these navicular cells are found in all conditions of intermediate cell proliferation.

The conditions in which the Navicular Cell are found, are as follows:

1. **Moderate oestrogen Deficiency**
   a. Secondary Amenorrhoea with low oestrogen as in
   b. Menopause
   c. Oligomenorrhoea

2. **Marked Progesterone Activity**
   i. In the second half of the menstrual cycle and pregnancy
   ii. Parental or oral administration of progesterone for therapeutic purposes
   iii. Persistent corpus luteum (in non pregnant women)

3. **Increased Androgen Activity**
   i. Post menopausal phase
   ii. Administration of androgen for therapeutic purposes
   iii. Hilus Cell Tumour of the Ovary

4. **Other conditions, where Deoderlein bacilli produce destruction of the mature layers of the vaginal epithelium**

Pundal (1966) remarked that the vaginal smear even with navicular cells in early pregnancy cannot be used as a reliable pregnancy test. In his series of cyto-hormonal evaluation of 6500 cases of pregnancy, he opined that early diagnosis of pregnancy was possible if:

a. Serial vaginal smears are reviewed in the particular cycle in which the patient becomes pregnant

Or

b. After an oestrogen test (Smith and Smith 1940). The administration of 5 – 10 milligrams of oestrogen for a few days prior to repeating a vaginal smear.

The results of this test show that the non pregnant female will react to it and show marked oestrogen effect, that is a high KPI; whereas in the pregnant women, there is no oestrogen effect (Wied 1957).

Although Papanicolaou stated that there is no striking difference in the pregnant and the non-pregnant navicular cell, Tarzano and Wachtel (1968) both observed that navicular cells of pregnancy appear to be smaller, oval and to have a much heavier membrane with oval and round nucleus while in a non-pregnant female in the luteal phase of the menstrual cycle, the navicular cells are larger, more navicular (boat shaped) with a fusiform nucleus. On the contrary, Shamim, Rizvi and Khan (1977) while working on hormonocytology of pregnancy found a characteristic boat shaped isolated navicular cell in the urinary sediment smear of a pregnant female, (as shown on page 11).

Hopman (1959) described ten criteria of pregnancy but the author himself later remarked that all these criteria may occur outside pregnancy and pregnancy can be present without these criteria. Therefore clinically colpocytogram has no particular value as a diagnostic tool in early pregnancy. Inspite of the limitations of vaginal cytology in normal pregnancy, the technique is very useful in screening the hormonal profile in patients with abnormal

pregnancy, such as abortion, as well as a reliable prognostic guide (Godefroy 1950, Pundal 1959, and Nesbitt 1961) and in the treatment of cases of abnormal pregnancy (Hochstaedt, 1960).

In most cases at the twelfth week of gestation, there is a transitory change in KPI, which increases 30 – 50% and EI up to 20% along with the appearance of a few parabasal cells. These changes usually revert to normal within a week, although there may be a a risk of abortion. Like others, Pundal (1958) believed the change to be due to the fact that the corpus luteum starts degenerating after the third month of gestation while the placenta has yet to reach its full hormonal activity. In cases where the KPI increases above 30%, it is considered abnormal (Nesbitt et al. 1961, De Neef 1965).

2. **Placental Phase of Pregnancy:**

a. The **Preterm period extends from the 12th to the 38th week of pregnancy**

Pundal and Van Meensel (1951) in their excellent monograph as well as in a subsequent publication, studied exhaustively the changes which occur in normal pregnancy until the onset of Labour. This phase included the second and third trimesters of pregnancy up to two weeks before Term (Pundal, 1959). Like the corpus luteum phase, this phase shows heavy exfoliation of intermediate cells with marked changes in KPI, EI, MV, under the effect of increased hormonal activity; this then continues as an uniform pattern of the normal pregnancy smear. (Microphotograph 4). This uniform pattern is also observed by Pundal 1959, Efstation, 1959, VonHaam 1961 and Shamim et al 1977.

1. a. Heavier exfoliation of the intermediate cells, with placard formation

   b. Cluster formation of the predominant navicular cells, which is the main element of the smear

2. Folding of cells, less accentuated

3. Curling of the squamous cells is the most striking phenomenon

4. Eosinophilic Index drops down gradually to below 5%

5. Karyopyknotic index decreases further to 10%

6. Marked shift in Maturation Index : to the mid zone in the Placental phase of Pregnancy, as shown below in Table 8.2.

Table 8.2

	$\longleftarrow$	
	$\longrightarrow$	
P	I	S
0.0	90 – 95	10 – 5

7. A certain percentage of the vaginal smears are cytolytic. The cytolysis typically starts in the first trimester and may increase in this phase. When the naked nuclei are above 50% then hormonal assessment becomes impossible. A single shot of intravaginal antibiotics, renders it cellular and thereafter an assessment can be carried out in the repeat smear

8. There is heavy growth of the Deoderlein bacilli, with which cytolysis increases.

9. Leucocytes, phagocytes are seen only when there is an infection in vagina particularly the T.V. infestation which is commonly seen in a multipara, who has previously suffered miscarriages

10. Cytolytic smears are mostly compatible with normal pregnancy smears and show no significance for the prenatal sex diagnosis (Pundal 1959 and VonHaam 1961). DeNeef (1965), Smolka and Soost (1965) and Koss (1968) have also reported similar changes during the second and third trimesters of pregnancy.

Most of the workers have reported the following modifications of the pregnancy smears in the placental phase of gestation -

1. Navicular Cell Type.

2. Cytolytic type

3. Inflammatory type

4. Oestrogenic type

Navicular cell type: The navicular cells predominate in normal pregnancy smears during the secondand third trimester. Wachtel (1968) described these cells as small oval shaped cells with markedly thickened boarders, delicate cytoplasm rich in glycogen with eccentrically placed oval or round vesicular nucleus. These cells have a tendency to cluster formation. Wachtel (1968) reported that the number and size of the individual cell clusters could be easily correlated with excretion of pregnandiol in the urine, and the progesterone effect in the smears can further be correlated with these, as shown below (Table 8.3)

The navicular cells, when stained by the Papanicolaou method appear pale bluish green. These cells are found in a variety of

Table 8.3: Shows comparative values of cell cluster with pregnandiol excretion in the urine under pro-gesterone effect

Progesterone effect in smear	Number of cells in individual cell cluster	Pregnandiol in the urine/24 Hrs
Good	10 – 15 Navicular cells	20 mgm/24 Hrs
Fair	5 – 9 Navicular cells	10–20 mgm/24 Hrs
Poor	0 – 1 Navicular cells	10 mgm/24 Hrs

conditions, hence their presence, as a rule, is not of diagnostic importance in pregnancy. It only indicates proliferation of the intermediate cells. However their shape, size and arrangement in the cluster appears to be of considerable significance in pregnancy with reference to the progesterone effect.

Cytolytic Smear Type: Cytolysis is observed quite often in normal pregnancy from the early phase (corpus luteum phase). It gradually increases in the placental phase accompanied by heavy growth of the Deoderlein bacilli. The excessively proliferated navicular cells, rich in glycogen, are a good source of nutrition for these bacilli. If there is any hormonal disturbance, then the Deoderlein bacilli in the cytolytic smear do not allow the intermediate cells to differentiate into superficial cells. When cytolysis persists, hormonal disturbance is not visible, following the normal phase (Pundal,1968).

Besides, this it has been demonstrated (Pundal and VanMeensel 1951, Pundal and Ost, E 1954; and Pundal 1957), that cytolysis has been observed in amenorrhoea, in the normal menstrual cycle, after castration as well as post administration of oestrogen, progesterone and androgen. The cytological picture is identical in these different conditions, which precludes the possibility of a definite hormonal diagnosis in the presence vaginal cytolysis.

The basic criteria defining marked cytolysis is the presence of naked nuclei of the same size and shaped more than 50% with predominant bacterial flora, i.e. Deoderlein bacilli. These criteria differentiate cytolysis from autolysis. It is thought that the predominance of progesterone is responsible for cytolysis. Teter (1968) has remarked that in disturbed hormonal states cytolysis may vanish. The mechanism of cytolysis is not well understood, and in some cases, with marked cytolysis, abnormal excretion values of oestrogen and pregnandiol have been reported by Godefroy (1955).

On the contrary, it has also been demonstrated experimentally in non pregnant women that oestrogen is unable to stop cytolysis in most cases (Wied 1953 and Pundal 1957). However, when cytolysis is marked the hormonal assessment based on the usual criteria of cellular indices is not possible, therefore Pundal suggested the rejection of hormonal assessment for cytolytic smears.

Dr. Ferin (1968) later advised that it is wise to inhibit cytolysis with a short course of local antibiotics which may be combined with a fungicide, particularly in women with a previous history of miscarriage, apparently due to endocrine disorders. We, in our routine practice, have only assessed the hormonal status of cytolytic cases in the repeat smear after the gynecologist has treated the patient with a local course of broad spectrum antibiotics. Thereafter the cytolytic smear is transformed into a normal cellular smear making cytohormonal evaluation possible. Nieburgs and Greenblatt (1948) believed that a cytolytic smear could have a significance for prenatal sex diagnosis. VonHaam (1961) and Pundal (1959) stated that cytolytic smears were compatible with normal pregnancies but could not be utilised for prenatal sex diagnosis.

Meisels (1968) mentioned that practically he always considered the two common pregnancy smears, that is navicular and cytolytics mears, to have the same prognostic significance. He thought that both smear types indicate normal hormonal balance in pregnancy. According to my observations in most of the cases, cytolytic smears indicated high level of progesterone, same as in the Navicular cell type which showed a good prognostic significance for a normally progressing pregnancy. Although Pundal (1959) had also mentioned that cytolytic smears during pregnancy indicate a good prognosis, yet it does not exclude some hormonal disturbances which in the intact smear would appear as an increase in EI and

KPI. Therefore he asked to reject these cases, as one cannot give a definite hormonal diagnosis on the routine criteria of cellular indices.

Ferin (1968) restated the challenge of correlating the vaginal smears and hormonal bioassays during pregnancy.He thought more refined techniques were needed for the measurement of the numerous estradiol and progesterone metabolites. He agreed with Engel (1965) who said that measurement carried out by an unspecified method for the total oestrogen, misses recognizing the fluctuations in the quantitative composition of the mixture even in cases where the total amount excreted remains the same.

Montalvo-Ruiz (1968) referred to the statement of Dr. Ferin, and said that although the question of the correlation between the vaginal smears and biological hormonal assays during the pregnancy had not been solved, but a great step forward was achieved as Brown could measure the levels of estrone, estradiol and estrone, produced by the placenta. Brown found that the placenta does not produce additional estriol up to the seventeenth week of gestation. It produces approximately 42% by the twentieth week, 53% by the thirtieth week and 60% at the end of gestation. Therefore now we cannot sustain the proposal expressed by Engel (1965).

Inflammatory Smear: This type of smear is more or less almost always associated with cervicitis, especially in a multipara. The study of Bret and co-worker(1959) showed that two-thirds of all the cases of vaginitis in pregnant women were caused by staphylococci and trichomonas vaginalis. Pundal (1959) observed that monilia fungal infection was found more frequently in pregnant women. All these infections are observed more in pregnant than in non-pregnant females. Such smears of infection show leucocytes, mucous and bacterial flora of a mixed variety. In addition, there is high KPI and pseudoeo-

sinophilia with perinuclear halo, karyorrhexis, karyolysis as well as dyskaryosis and phagocytosis in severe infection (VonHaam 1961). In our series, we have observed dysplastic changes with phagocytosis, if there is trichomonas infestation, which is occasionally responsible for early abortions.

Birtch (1961) reported only 10% inflammatory smears while VonHaam (1961) found 35% infection in their pregnant patients. Ruiz (1968) recorded 30% infection in his cases, while Rahman and Zaman (1963) from Karachi have reported trichomonas vaginalis 5% in pregnant and 15% in non pregnant females. Further they could find moniliasis 18% in pregnant 10% in nonpregnant. Shamim Khan and Rizvi (1977) found the following incidence of infection among the 130 pregnant women in their vaginal, vulval and urinary sediment smears, shown in Table 8.3, where it is seen that urinary sediment smears were free of specific infections.

Table 8.4: Incidence of Infection–Comparative Values (Shamim; Khan and Rizvi 1977)

Types of Infection	Vaginal		Vulval		Urinary Sediment Smears
Non specific	32	12.6	25	9.8	1.9
Fungal	6	2.3	4	1.5	0
Trichomonas Vag.	2	0.7	2	0.7	0

In cases of vaginal infection,local treatment with antibiotics and antifungal drugs should be instituted; thereafter, repeat smear assessment postclearance of infection should be checked for the presence of abnormalities such as dysplasia and anaplasia.Further VonHaam (1961) reported that cellular atypia in trichomonas infection creates diagnostic difficulties. This problem in a multipara is suggestive of an etiologic relationship of the infection with cancer cervix. Fiftyfour authors after discussion, in the first symposium on "Cancer Cytology during Pregnancy" (1959) agreed that cancer occurs on an average, at 0.02 percent or in one out of every 5000 pregnancies, and that approximately 1.6% of patients with cancer of cervix were pregnant. It was suggested that all pregnant patients should therefore be screened for cervical carcinoma.

Oestrogenic Type of Smear: The reported incidence of the oestrogenic type of smear in pregnancy is 15% (VonHaam 1961). This type of vaginal smear contains a few navicular cells without characteristic clumping. These smears are dominated by acidophilic and pyknotic superficial cells, typical of preovulatory smear type. These are observed in the first six weeks of gestation. If thispersists, it indicates serious hormonal abnormalities (VonHaam 1961).

b. **"At Term" period 38 – 40 weeks of gestation shows At Term Pregnancy Smear Pattern:**

Pundal and Lichtfus (1959) **observed** that the uniform preterm pattern of pregnancy is modified in the last two weeks before term on account of a drop in the hormonal levels; this they labeled as "at term".

Many workers, Pundal (1959), Ruiz (1965), Malek (1967), on the basis of the above observations, introduced the concept that vaginal smear is of practical value at the end of pregnancy. Further it was noted that the drop in the hormonal levels at "at term" brings about spontaneous labour within 5 days (Pundal 1959, Ruiz 1965 and Malek 1967, and Pandit et al. 1986). Hence "at term" changes are important to predict the onset of labor.

The "at term" smear is characterized by the following changes, as shown in the Microphotograph 5 (Shamim, Khan and Rizvi)

1. Breakup of large clusters of navicular cells into smaller at "at term" or isolated cells at "near term", without changes in shape and staining qualities of cells
2. The Karyopyknotic as well as the acidophilic indices rise to 30–50%. This peak is

shortlived, subsequently it changes and both the KPI and the EI disappear
3. There is loss of curling, folding and crowding and thus more discrete intermediate cells are seen
4. The intermediate cells are mostly replaced by the superficial cells, which are also discrete, flat polygonal cells and resemble the proliferative phase of the menstrual cycle

Pundal and Lichtfus (1959) reported that vaginal cytology should permit one to determine with an accuracy greater than 90%, on whether the pregnancy is "at term". They further mention that as long as the pregnancy smear is of the "before term" type, post maturity can be confidently excluded, even though gestation has long exceeded the calculated chronologic term. On the other hand if the smear is of the "postpartum" type, the pregnancy requires termination immediately, since it indicates a serious danger to the foetus. In their opinion, a smear "at term" is a safe guide to the choice of artificial induction of labour. They further mention that if the smear is of the preterm type, then the induction of labour even in cases where the calculated term is complete, will fail; whereas the smear being of the "at term" type ensures that the induction of labor will be successful at the first trial in 95 percent of cases.

Pundal's work stimulated Birtch (1961) to undertake a similar study in pregnancy to observe "at term" changes. He obtained 19,000 vaginal smears for this study from approximately 9000 private patients of four different obstetricians, practicing during a period (1949–1959) of 10 years. In his study Birtch could not confirm the opinion of Pundal that the assessment of vaginal smear is of practical value to determine the end of pregnancy, although he followed the Pundal's technique.

According to Birtch (1961), the initiation of progressive labour has not yet been conclusively demonstrated. The theory that the fall in hormonal level is the "initiating cause of Labour" is not universally accepted. He found in his observations, that patients with poor obstetric history (repeated still births) showed that foetus in most cases expired first, while the placenta continued to produce sex hormones. Hence it may be concluded that cytologicstudies are not helpful to predict the onset of labour. Birtch finally concluded that his studies suggested that vaginal cytology may offer the obstetricians under certain varied conditions and at various times during pregnancy, a simple and inexpensive means of evaluating the course of pregnancy.

The entire predicament of diagnosis by ante-partum smears continues to remains uncertain. In addition to Birtch, Abrams and Abrams (1962), Hammad (1965), Meisels (1966) and Jung (1969), took a less favourable view. Handman, Schwalenberg and Efstation(1962) along with Wachtel (1969), denied that these changes occur regularly in a significant number of cases at the end of pregnancy. They further emphasized that prediction of onset of labour from these criteria is misleading. On the other hand, according to large number of workers it was found to be a useful parameter for assessing the approximate date of birth (Dehnhard, 1973, 1975, Lichtfus 1964, Miklaw 1961, Pundal 1952, 1959 Steinhoff, 1975,Ortner 1977, Pandit et al 1986}

Malek (1967) also discussed that the biologic preparation of labor is a complex process, principally based on a shift in the oestrogen–progesterone relationship. This hormonal shift can be observed adequately from the criteria of onset of labour. Study by means of cytology, hormonal assessment was used as an index for determining biological preparation of spontaneous labour "at term". The cytologic evaluation in these cases provided an estimate of the quality of hormonal preparation of labour. In this way the cytologic examination helps in deter-mining further clinical treatment, that is, expectation or induction of uterine contraction.

Ortner from his work of 1974–75 concluded-

a. In cytohormonal evaluation if the cell picture at the end of pregnancy (chronologically) was preterm, then a postmaturity syndrome could be excluded with a probability of 95 to 100%.

b. Further he reported that in the cell picture "at term" an entire palette of monitoring parameters requires to be employed, since signs of post maturity appear in 1 to 10% of cases. Moreover the "at term" smear permits approximate determination of the date of birth and one can consider induction of labor in these cases, since the probability of immaturity of the foetus is only 0 to 5%.

c. In Ortner's cases(1974–75), spontaneous delivery took place in 86.4% within the next five days when the smear predicted the start of labor.

Later Ortner (1977) attributed great importance to vaginal cytology at the end of pregnancy. This method allowed him to select from the large group of patients with diagnostic problems of "at term", those who required more sophisticated monitoring methods.

Ortner et al. (1977) used the same cytologic finding "preterm", "at term" and "post term" (similar to the other workers) for clinical assessment. He paid special attention to eosinophilia and pyknosis and thus supplemented the subjective qualitative criteria of the cytologic diagnosis with objective criteria. Thereafter a linear discriminant analysis (Weber E-1972) was subsequently performed and a function to separate "pre term" and "at term" was carried out. Using the analysis at variance, it was found that it yields a true separation of the two collectives "preterm" and "at term".

The results obtained by the above method of evaluation indicate:

1. Special attention should be paid to eosin-

hormonal cytodiagnosis, as far as the complexity of these particular hormonal activities can allow of such a differential diagnosis.

The classification described in the "Symposium on Hormonal Cytology" by Pundal 1968 is as follows:

1. **Smear of Superficial cell types**

   a. **MIa:** Mostly flat or slightly folded cells but without clusters.

   b. **MIb:** Mostly folded but single cells.

   c. **MIc:** Folded cells in clusters.

2. **Smears of Intermediate cell type**

   a. **MII:** The usual, intermediate of type of cells, which are the predominant elements of the smear. Parabasal cells are absent.

3. Smears of the parabasal or sub atrophic type

   a. **M III:** Intermediate and parabasal cells.

4. **Smears of the completely atrophic type (MVI)**

5. **The androgenic smear type (MA)**

6. **The cytolytic smear type (MC)**

7. **Mixed smear types**

   This classification is schematic, based mainly upon the predominant cell type except for some particular cell changes independent of the cell type. It usually permits hormonal analysis with the exception of majority of cases with mixed smears (Complex Adreno–Cortical Activity).

   For the menopausal women, cytohormonal norms were suggested by Meisels (1966) and Stone et al (1967). The cytohormonal readings by Meisels were based on the differential count of vaginal part of VCE (Vaginal Cervical Endocervical on a single slide) smears, stained by Papanicolaou method. This differential count included 5 types of squamous cells, assigned a specific value, which is as follows:

   i. Superficial Eosinophilic Cell – 1.0

   ii. Superficial Cyanophilic Cell – 0.8

   iii. Large Intermediate Cell – 0.6

   iv. Small Intermediate Cell – 0.5

   v. Parabasal Cell –0.0

   Percentage of each cell was multiplied by its value and the results added. The sum (without decimal) were called as **Oestrogenic Value.**

   The oestrogenic value, calculated on the basis of differential count was later labelled as Maturation value (MV) of Frost. Meisels in 1967, suggested to reduce the number of cell types to three, with little change in the value, as described by Frost in the Terminology symposium (1958).

   The change was as follows (1) Superficial Eosinophilic Pyknotic Cell = 1.0, Intermediate = 0.5, and Basal Cell = 0.0.

   The advantage of the Oestrogenic Value is that like MV it could easily be submitted for statistical analysis.

   Meisels in 1966 published a report on cytohormonal evaluation of 5920 menopausal women who could fulfil the following additional criteria:

a. Adequate clinical information regarding the age, date of last menstrual period, Pelvic Surgery or radiotherapy (if given)

b. Technically a good smear (after taking precautions)

c. No marked inflammatory changes with impaired morphology of vaginal cells were observed of Trichomonas Vaginalis infection or Moniliasis.

d. No hormonal treatment was given three months prior to the collection of smears.

The observations of the studies of Meisels (1966) revealed that:

1. The age distribution indicated a normal pattern between the ages of 45 to 64 years in 70% of the cases, and there was a variation in the age of onset of menopause.

2. It was found that mean oestrogenic values were quite comparable with age and time elapsed since menopause.

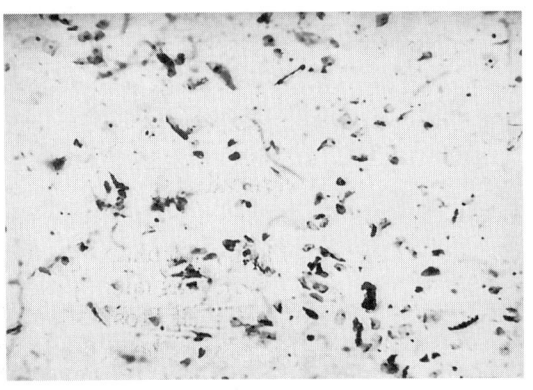

Microphotograph 3C: 1st Trimester pattern
Urinary Sediment
Smear
(Pap. X70)

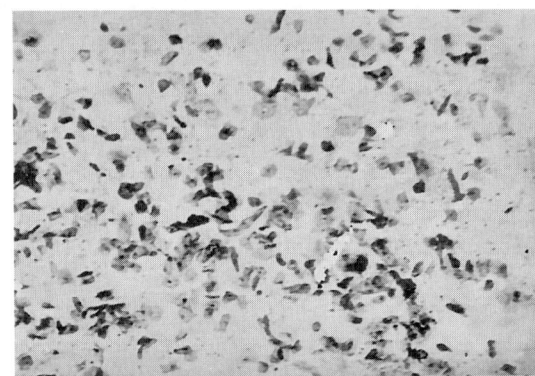

Microphotograph 4C: "Mid Term" pattern
Urinary Sediment
Smear
(Pap. X70)

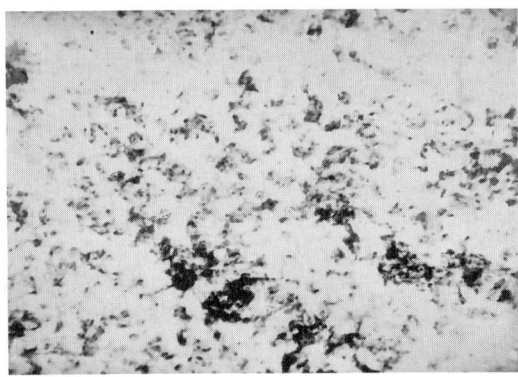

Microphotograph 4A: "Mid Term" Pattern
Vaginal Smear
(Pap. X70)

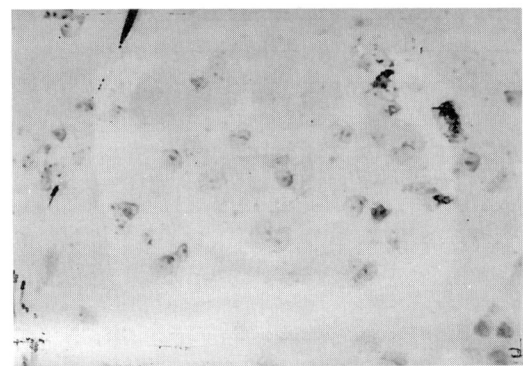

Microphotograph 5A: "At Term" Pattern
Vaginal Smear
(Pap. X70)

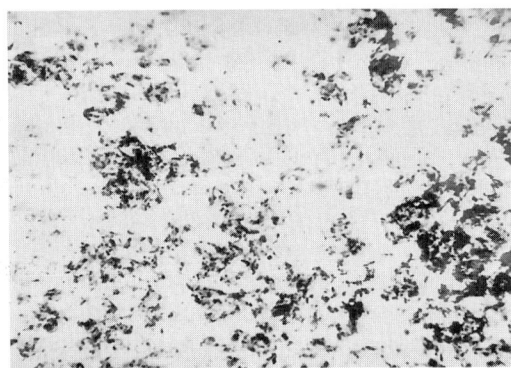

Microphotograph 4B: "Mid Term" Pattern
Vulval Smear
(Pap. X70)

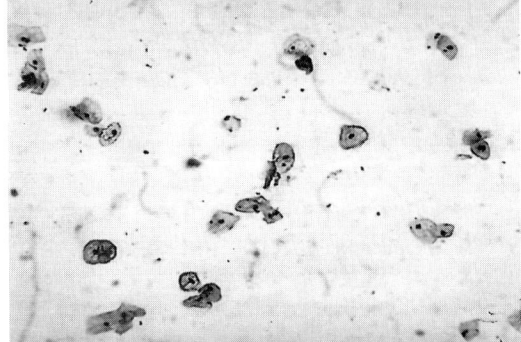

Microphotograph 5B: "At Term" Pattern
Vulval Smear
(Pap. X70)

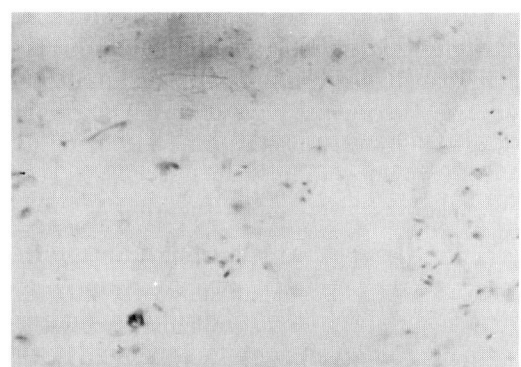

Microphotography 5C: "At Term" pattern
Urinary Sediment
Smear (Pap. X70)

POSTNATAL HORMONAL CYTOLOGY

During the discussion in the "Symposium on Hormonal Cytology During Pregnancy" (1959), all the deliberators unanimously agreed with the postpartum cytological observation of Pundal and Van Meensel (1951). They recognized the immediate postpartum changes, i.e. the Postpartum Pattern, similar in all women, changes which last until the tenth day after delivery. The appearance of the second or remaining postpartum period changes depend on whether the woman is lactating or not. This second phase is from the tenth day until the return of menstrual cycle in the sixth week (or 4 – 8 weeks) in the non-lactating women and up to 4 to 9 months in the lactating women.

During this period a few morphologic entities with a distinctive appearance have been described in the hormonocytology of the postpartum period, e.g. "Lactation cells", "Postpartum cells", Postnatal cells. These descriptions mentioned in the past should be distinguished from parabasal and small intermediate cells of Papanicolaou (1933), and Pundal (1951), respectively.

Immediate Postpartum Period: In this phase vaginal smears resemble the castrated or menopausal smear with blood and pus cells in the first few days, followed quickly by a large number of histocytes. The Navicular cells disappear and are replaced by a large number of modified parabasal cells for which in 1954 Papanicolaou coined the name "Postpartum" cells.

These "postpartum cells"were first described by Papanicolaou and Traut. These were oval or round, mostly like the large parabasal cells, characterized by thick prominent margins, partly pyknotic nuclei and with vacuolated bluish cytoplasm. But occasionally these were eosinophilic with pyknotic nuclei.

In the second phase, after delivery, post partum cells assumed the configuration of normal parabasal cells which was due to decrease in glycogen in the cytoplasm (Nyklicek 1959). Later Boschann (1968) described these postpartum cells in great detail.

These postpartum cells described by Boschann(1968), are a transitive form between the navicular and the parabasal cells according to their shape, size and staining. Their main character is their distinct light refracting border with the cyanophilic cytoplasm which is darker than in the navicular cells and brighter than in the parabasal cells. Histochemically, the cytoplasm is rich in glycogen, and vacuolization can also be found. The nucleus is not as dense in the chromatin structure as in the parabasal cells but is usually more dense than in the navicular cells. Nuclei can be vesicular or pyknotic and spoon shaped or rod like or leaf like in shape as it is found in the intermediate cells during pregnancy.

These postpartum cells originate from the outer parabasal layer. This layer become very hypertrophic during pregnancy and exfoliates after delivery. Boschann found these cells in one third of the cases on the fifth day of delivery both in lactating and nonlactating women, while Ruiz (1968) mentioned that he could find postpartum cells in 50% of his cases on the 5th or 6th day after delivery. Postpartum cells disappear on the woman's

In this study of 5920 cases,Meisels found that an appreciable number of patients retain a cytologically detectable oestrogenic activity far into old age. He determined the hormone value range during menopause and established the criteria for selecting menopausal patients eligible for hormonal treatment on basis of the oestrogenic values. He found three levels of oestrogenic activity in the menopause, which were as follows:-

a. Absent or Very Low – (EV 0 – 49) Decreasing in value gradually, in about half of the patients, with increasing years of menopause. In 21% of the cases, complete atrophy (EV 0) was observed.

b. Moderate Value – (EV 50 - 64) was found in 40% cases, who maintained it throughout life.

c. High Value – (EV 65–Over) 10% cases only, who carried it far into the old age.

These results confirm the work of others, who reported persistent oestrogenic activity in the menopausal period (Struthers – 1956, Allende 1950, Masukawa, 1960, Ruiz 1964, Muth 1960, Peters, 1960).

In 1956, Struthers could find only 20.1% of atrophic smears in the group of 353 menopausal patients, which is almost exactly the same finding as observed later by Meisels in 1966. He further observed that even after 25 years of menopause, atrophic smears did not exceed 40%.

Later Joshi, Saraiya and Fernandes (1971) studied cytology in 475 cases of menopause, attending the cytology clinic of Cama and Albless Hospital, Mumbai from December 1969 to Ju;ly 1971. Among these inflammatory 52.6% and abnormal 12.14% smears were found. Cytohormonal evaluation was possible in 110 cases out of 429 with natural menopause. Out of these 429 cases50.9% showed considerable oestrogenic activity and maturity, which is comparable to the finding of the other worker. It was observed that there was a gradual decline of oestrgenic activity in the vaginal smears with the increasing duration of the menopause, further they found that urocytogram was not suitable for hormonal study in these cases. As far as estimation of hormones was concerned, there was higher urinary oestrogen levels in the earlier years after the menopause and with more mature cells. They could estimate 24 hrs total urinary oestrogen in 52 cases according to the Brown flurometric method (1968). Abnormal smears were rare in asymptomatic and in cases with prolapsed of the uterus.

Stone et al (1967) also reported oestrogen like effect in the vaginal smears of 340 chronically ill postmenopausal women, aged 40 years to 98 years. The study of KPI, MI and MV was carried out in those women who were menopausal for at least two years. In this group, the longest period of menopause was 48 years. The smears were collected from the lateral wall of vagina and stained with standard Papanicolaou staining technique. Patients receiving oestrogen therapy, patients with malignancy and patients who failed to respond to vaginitis treatment were excluded from this study. Stone et al modified the oestrogenic value calculation that all the superficial cells (both oesinophilic and cyanophilic) were arbitrarily valued at 0.9. Therefore now the range of value (maximum) was MV–90, which could be compared with oestrogenic effect. The interpretation of MV requires to be matched with the age and patient history.

The results in healthy women showed that the predominance of low values (0–49) was 41% during first decade of menopause and as high as 82% in the 5th decade of menopause. The percentage of women with high maturation value (65–90) remained at approximately the same level, that is, 8.9% through the first 30 years of postmenopause, then dropped to 3% in the fourth decade and 0% in the fifth decade of menopause.

Stone et al (1967) carried out work in the chronically ill postmenopausal patients. The KPI, MI and MV indices were used in this study to correlate oestrogen like effect with

hormonal cytodiagnosis, as far as the complexity of these particular hormonal activities can allow of such a differential diagnosis.

The classification described in the "Symposium on Hormonal Cytology" by Pundal 1968 is as follows:

1. **Smear of Superficial cell types**

    a. **MIa:** Mostly flat or slightly folded cells but without clusters.

    b. **MIb:** Mostly folded but single cells.

    c. **MIc:** Folded cells in clusters.

2. **Smears of Intermediate cell type**

    a. **MII:** The usual, intermediate of type of cells, which are the predominant elements of the smear. Parabasal cells are absent.

3. Smears of the parabasal or sub atrophic type

    a. **M III:** Intermediate and parabasal cells.

4. **Smears of the completely atrophic type (MVI)**

5. **The androgenic smear type (MA)**

6. **The cytolytic smear type (MC)**

7. **Mixed smear types**

    This classification is schematic, based mainly upon the predominant cell type except for some particular cell changes independent of the cell type. It usually permits hormonal analysis with the exception of majority of cases with mixed smears (Complex Adreno–Cortical Activity).

    For the menopausal women, cytohormonal norms were suggested by Meisels (1966) and Stone et al (1967). The cytohormonal readings by Meisels were based on the differential count of vaginal part of VCE (Vaginal Cervical Endocervical on a single slide) smears, stained by Papanicolaou method. This differential count included 5 types of squamous cells, assigned a specific value, which is as follows:

    i. Superficial Eosinophilic Cell – 1.0

    ii. Superficial Cyanophilic Cell – 0.8

    iii. Large Intermediate Cell – 0.6

    iv. Small Intermediate Cell – 0.5

    v. Parabasal Cell –0.0

    Percentage of each cell was multiplied by its value and the results added. The sum (without decimal) were called as **Oestrogenic Value**.

    The oestrogenic value, calculated on the basis of differential count was later labelled as Maturation value (MV) of Frost. Meisels in 1967, suggested to reduce the number of cell types to three, with little change in the value, as described by Frost in the Terminology symposium (1958).

    The change was as follows (1) Superficial Eosinophilic Pyknotic Cell = 1.0, Intermediate = 0.5, and Basal Cell = 0.0.

    The advantage of the Oestrogenic Value is that like MV it could easily be submitted for statistical analysis.

    Meisels in 1966 published a report on cytohormonal evaluation of 5920 menopausal women who could fulfil the following additional criteria:

a. Adequate clinical information regarding the age, date of last menstrual period, Pelvic Surgery or radiotherapy (if given)

b. Technically a good smear (after taking precautions)

c. No marked inflammatory changes with impaired morphology of vaginal cells were observed of Trichomonas Vaginalis infection or Moniliasis.

d. No hormonal treatment was given three months prior to the collection of smears.

The observations of the studies of Meisels (1966) revealed that:

1. The age distribution indicated a normal pattern between the ages of 45 to 64 years in 70% of the cases, and there was a variation in the age of onset of menopause.

2. It was found that mean oestrogenic values were quite comparable with age and time elapsed since menopause.

ABORTIONS

Corpus luteum phase: (First Trimester)

1. Incidence of Abortions:

Gaudefroy (1959) reported that the incidence of spontaneous abortion was approximately 15% of all pregnancies, of which 6 to 7% were due to endocrine dysfunction.

a. **Early Abortion:** This is the most common disorder of early pregnancy. However, there are certain cell types which are observed in the cases of very early pregnancy, subsequently terminating in abortion at the time of expected menstruation. These cells are highly active in appearance, the nuclei are large with prominent nucleoli and the cytoplasm is often scanty and ill defined. These cells morphologically are undifferentiated and present themselves as a large sheet, small clumps or as an isolated cell. On account of their active nuclei these cells give the false suspicion of malignancy but actually are the embryonic cells of early abortion (Nelson 1967). According to statistics available in America, Nelson found that foetal death rate per 1000 live birth in USA in 1964 was 16.4% and the average gestation period in these cases was over 20 weeks. Hertig (1967) reported 28.5% abortion rate for a group of women, who had missed their first menstrual period and had an immediate (non clinical) or delayed (clinical) abortion. Iffy (1965) had also observed that the majority of gestations which eventually ended as early spontaneous abortion were actually cases which soon after fertilization were followed by bleeding at the time of expected menstruation.

Nelson (1967) had compared the vaginal pool smears of the known cases of early abortion with the histological sections of early known human pregnancies and cytologic preparation of chick embryos to confirm that these active suspicious looking cells were found in cases of early (non clinical) or late (clinical) abortion mostly occurred at the time of menstrual flow. This report will be helpful for a cytopathologist in avoiding the false suspicion of malignancy, while reporting on Early Abortion cases.

b. **Threatened Abortion:** Dellipiane (1959) mentioned the characteristics of Threatened Aborton in the first trimester, at the "Symposium on Hormonal Cytology during Pregnancy" as an eosinophilic index greater than 35% along with navicular cells, some RBC, abundant mucous and a predominance of the superficial cells.

Von Haam (1961) stated that the most important indication of Threatened Abortion is an increase in karyopyknotic and eosinophilic indices with concomitant reduction in the navicular cells and their decreased inclination to form clumps.

These above findings in the vaginal smears provide valuable information, if the prior smears of these pregnant women were normal from the onset of pregnancy, but it was of no value in those who had persistently oestrogenic smear from the beginning. Thus the Threatened Abortion in the first trimester, poses achallenge as to whether steps should be taken to expedite abortion or to conserve the pregnancy. In such cases, hormonal bioassays are a useful tool to diagnose hormonal disorders of early pregnancy as well as to regulate the therapy. A review of a significant number of statistical reports teaches us that the biochemical assays are of real significance only when these are markedly abnormal (Klopper 1963) and if these could be repeated several times. In routine practice, biochemical assays can only be carried out in a well established laboratory, having sophisticated equipment. The tests are expensive and the privilege of few affording individuals. Conversely, cytodiagnosis is simple, easy, quick, atraumatic as well as an economical procedure. It can be repeated as many times as required. It is the best control test not only to follow the course of pregnancy but also to distinguish the effect of hormonal therapy in cases of disturbed pregnancy.

Gaudefroy (1959) reported in a study of 1450 pregnancy smears that out of 1176 cases (without a history of previous abortion) with normal cytohormonal pattern, 0.77 percent aborted. While Pundal (1957) had reported 0.59 percent abortion rate out of 3393 cases of normally progressing pregnancies. Thus 99.23% and 99.41%respectively in Gaudefroy's and Pundal's cases delivered live babies. Therefore they concluded that the above finding showed that there is little chance of abortion in the normally progressing pregnancy and one can easily predict with the help of cytology those cases which could go to Term Pregnancy.

Birtch (1961) also reported that vaginal cytogram in a pregnant female is a highly reliable and sensitive method for forecasting the outcome of Pregnancy.

Nesbitt (1961) proved that the vaginal cytogram indicates hormonal inadequacy before it can be detected by the hormonal assay.

Osmond – Clarke and Murray (1963) reported that while working on recurrent abortions cases, they found a few cases of abnormal smear pattern, in which urinary excretion of hormones was found normal, thus they also suggested that colpocytogram was a more sensitive indicator than the biochemical assays.

MacRae (1967) has also mentioned that colpocytogram is a truer guide for the hormonal status of a female than the hormonal assays, while working on the correlation between the vaginal cytology and urinary hormone assay in pregnancy.

Criteria of Hormonal Disturbance in Threatened Abortion:

1. Disappearance of Navicular cells
2. Gradual disappearance of Intermediate cells
3. Loss of curling and folding
4. Appearance of cyanophilic and eosinophilic superficial cells in considerable number
5. Increase in Karyopyknotic Index – above 15 to 25%
6. Increase in Eosinophilic Index – above 5 to 10%

Gaudefroy (1959) has reported that he found an opportunity to cytologically observe 178 cases of threatened abortion, who were under oestrogen treatment. The details of the cases were (Table 9.1A):

1. Cytoprognostic: Normal smear – Errors = 2.63% (limit 0.06 – 13.1%)
2. Error: abnormal smear = 15.07% (limit of 9.77 to 21.85%)

Statistical significance between the two groups with regard to the outcome of pregnancy t = 2.16; 0.02 < P < 0.05 (Judicial limit). From this table it is seen that in cases where the pregnancy smears were normal, 97.3% living children were delivered, including a few premature babies; while in

Table 9.1A: Details of 178 cases of Threatened Abortion under Estrogen Treatment (Gaudefroy 1959)

		Abortions		Child Birth		
		Living Ovum	Blighted Ovum	Normal	Premature	
					N	Abn
THREATENED	Normal (38) Cyto Hormonal Smear	0	1	34	3	0
ABORTIONS	Abnormal (140) Cytohormonal Smears	1	21	95	20	3
Total	178	1	22	129	23	3

In this study of 5920 cases,Meisels found that an appreciable number of patients retain a cytologically detectable oestrogenic activity far into old age. He determined the hormone value range during menopause and established the criteria for selecting menopausal patients eligible for hormonal treatment on basis of the oestrogenic values. He found three levels of oestrogenic activity in the menopause, which were as follows:-

a. Absent or Very Low – (EV 0 – 49) Decreasing in value gradually, in about half of the patients, with increasing years of menopause. In 21% of the cases, complete atrophy (EV 0) was observed.

b. Moderate Value – (EV 50 - 64) was found in 40% cases, who maintained it throughout life.

c. High Value – (EV 65–Over) 10% cases only, who carried it far into the old age.

These results confirm the work of others, who reported persistent oestrogenic activity in the menopausal period (Struthers – 1956, Allende 1950, Masukawa, 1960, Ruiz 1964, Muth 1960, Peters, 1960).

In 1956, Struthers could find only 20.1% of atrophic smears in the group of 353 menopausal patients, which is almost exactly the same finding as observed later by Meisels in 1966. He further observed that even after 25 years of menopause, atrophic smears did not exceed 40%.

Later Joshi, Saraiya and Fernandes (1971) studied cytology in 475 cases of menopause, attending the cytology clinic of Cama and Albless Hospital, Mumbai from December 1969 to Ju;ly 1971. Among these inflammatory 52.6% and abnormal 12.14% smears were found. Cytohormonal evaluation was possible in 110 cases out of 429 with natural menopause. Out of these 429 cases50.9% showed considerable oestrogenic activity and maturity, which is comparable to the finding of the other worker. It was observed that there was a gradual decline of oestrgenic activity in the vaginal smears with the increasing duration of the menopause, further they

found that urocytogram was not suitable for hormonal study in these cases. As far as estimation of hormones was concerned, there was higher urinary oestrogen levels in the earlier years after the menopause and with more mature cells. They could estimate 24 hrs total urinary oestrogen in 52 cases according to the Brown flurometric method (1968). Abnormal smears were rare in asymptomatic and in cases with prolapsed of the uterus.

Stone et al (1967) also reported oestrogen like effect in the vaginal smears of 340 chronically ill postmenopausal women, aged 40 years to 98 years. The study of KPI, MI and MV was carried out in those women who were menopausal for at least two years. In this group, the longest period of menopause was 48 years. The smears were collected from the lateral wall of vagina and stained with standard Papanicolaou staining technique. Patients receiving oestrogen therapy, patients with malignancy and patients who failed to respond to vaginitis treatment were excluded from this study. Stone et al modified the oestrogenic value calculation that all the superficial cells (both oesinophilic and cyanophilic) were arbitrarily valued at 0.9. Therefore now the range of value (maximum) was MV–90, which could be compared with oestrogenic effect. The interpretation of MV requires to be matched with the age and patient history.

The results in healthy women showed that the predominance of low values (0–49) was 41% during first decade of menopause and as high as 82% in the 5th decade of menopause. The percentage of women with high maturation value (65–90) remained at approximately the same level, that is, 8.9% through the first 30 years of postmenopause, then dropped to 3% in the fourth decade and 0% in the fifth decade of menopause.

Stone et al (1967) carried out work in the chronically ill postmenopausal patients. The KPI, MI and MV indices were used in this study to correlate oestrogen like effect with

diabetes, heart and circulatory diseases, cirrhosis of the liver, renal diseases, central nervous system disorders and with Digitalis therapy. The KPI, MI and MV indices served as good indicators of oestrogen activity. The results of the above were as follows:

1. No rise in oestrogen activity in the vaginal epithelium of diabetics who were on therapy and diet control.

   On the other hand Magie (1967) reported that in women with atleastone year of menopause, aged 44 years to 80 years who were clinically diabetic, (with impaired glucose tolerance test), there was increased oestrogen level in the vaginal smears of two third of patients. The endometrial biopsy of these cases revealed glandular hyperplasia and endometrial carcinoma in one third cases as a result of high levels of oestrogenfor a prolonged period. In these cases, the sequence of impaired carbohydrate metabolism leads to excess oestrogen production which is responsible for the endometrial pathology.

2. In cirrhosis of the liver, there was no evidence of increased oestrogen,although it has been generally believed that the conjugation of oestrogen is impaired in this disease leading to an increase in the level of the oestrogen hormone.

3. In rural patients with similar diseases, lower values were observed, but since the number of cases were few, a confirmation of this was not possible.

4. Patients with cardiovascular and central nervous system disease, arthritis, cases with fractures, none of them showed any abnormal level of oestrogen activity.

5. Patients on digitalis therapy exhibited increased oestrogen like effect confirming the report of other investigators (Brunori 1965, Charles 1966 and Navab et al 1965). This reaction is explained by the similarity in the molecular structure of the active principle of digitals glycoside (glucose) and that of oestrone. On the contrary Gorden et

al found no increase in maturation values in their study (1966) in digitalis therapy patients.

6. The incidence of vaginitis was high in postmenopausal women but a marked decrease was found in digitalis therapy cases.

The relatively low incidence of atrophy and the finding of an adequate maturation of the vaginal epithelium in the majority of cases, reported by all the workers in this field, indicates that oestrogen treatment in menopausal women should not be used indiscriminately. An accurate cytohormonal evaluation should always be carried out before and after treatment for the assessment of the effect of therapy.

Investigations of Papaniculaou (1933) to date and the reports of large numbers of workers in this field have proved the value of vaginal cytology in the assessment of endocrine activity. Papanicolaou in 1945, while working on detection of cancer cells in the urinary sediment smears discovered that significant cytologic changes could be noted much more readily in these than in the vaginal smears. Thus his attention was diverted to the study of urinary sediment smears (catheterised specimens) in pregnant females (1947). He found that this simple rapid cytologic technique can easily be utilised in pregnancy, as morphologically cells show great similarity with that of the vaginal cells.

Later Del-Castillo et al (1948-49) also described that urinary sediment smears show similar variations of hormonal activity as in vaginal smears and subsequent studies of Lencioni 1963–69 demonstrated the usefulness of this technique in hormonal cytology.

In 1965–66 Delcastillo et al discovered a similar cycle in the cells exfoliated from the inner surface of labia minora in child bearing age and prepubertal girls. He performed this investigation also in menopausal and pregnant women and proved that labia minora smear (nymphocytogram) was equally an accurate index of ovarian activity.

found that the accuracy of prediction which was 81% in pre-oestrogen phase increased to 90% in the post oestrogen phase. The above results suggest that the diagnostic as well as prognostic accuracy of the oestrogen test on the cytohormonal smears is high in normal as well as in abnormal smears. Thus this is a reliable useful test in routine clinical practice.

It is said that oestrogen stimulates the production of progesterone from the placenta (Smith, Smith and Schiller 1941) on the basis of which Pundal et al (1951) proposed the administration of oestrogen and progesterone together in cases of threatened abortion.

In the Symposium on "Hormonal Cytology During Pregnancy" (1959) many workers presented their opinion regarding the signs of abortion in a vaginal smear.

Ramos (1959) suggested that an abundance of superficial cells (more than 40%) and a scarcity of navicular cells are signs of threatened abortion due to progesterone deficiency.

Dellipiane(1959) reported that an eosinophilic index higher than 35% may be considered abnormal. Pundal (1959) mentioned that in his experience, an eosinophilic index above 50% in several smears, taken at intervals of few days predicted poor prognosis, in a pregnancy that was older than 3 months.

Almost all the workers in this field have conferred importance to increasing cornification (that is, high KPI and EI) in the vaginal smears as a sign of threatened abortion. On the basis of KPI (cornification), Birtch (1961) attempted to classify the smears of threatened abortion into three categories:-

Mild, Moderate and Marked

1. **Mild:** Smears show scattered cornification along with an increase in KPI, EI along with a concomitant reduction in the navicular

cells and their inclination for clustering.

2. **Moderate:** Vaginal smear shows a 30-40 percent increase in KPI, with a high EI and a low count of isolated or small groups of navicular cells. In these cases it is advised to initiate hormonal treatment (oestrogen therapy) as advised by Smith and Smith (1946). These cases will revert to a normal pregnancy smear with or, occasionally, without therapy.

Bourg and coworker (1953), Pundal and Gaudefroy (1959), Birtch (1961), and VonHaam (1961) confirmed that vaginal cytology is a good prognostic method to assess the efficiency or inefficiency of hormonal therapy. Gaudefroy even showed that when the ovum is dead, following oestrogen administration, a postpartum or a post abortion type of smear is seen.

Birtch (1961) carried out a study of 1851 patients over a period of 3 years to evaluate the different oestrogen therapy regimens (Smith and Smith 1946), popular in the treatment of threatened abortion.

His view after this review was as follows:

  i. Patients with deficient type of smears had 4 ½ times the greater chance of abortion than those who had normal or "good" smear patterns.

 ii. Administration of stilbestrol in the amount recommended, certainly did not reduce the incidence of abortion in patients with a moderate deficiency type of smear. On the contrary,Pundal (1959) Gaudefroy (1959) Kaufman (1969) and Rizvi et al (1978) advised administration of the hormone in moderate cases which was helpful in reducing the incidence of abortion; in other words, the salvage rate was increased (Osmond–Clarke et al. (1963).

3. **Marked:** Most of the cells, in these untreated cases were cornified cells with a high KPI followed by the appearance of

parabasal cells. Even in cases of disturbed pregnancy, when stilbesterol treatment resulted in an increase in the mature superficial cells (high KPI), it indicates nonviability of the foetus. Later appearance of parabasal cells leading to regressive smear indicated that abortion was inevitable. The persistence or increase in parabasal cells confirmed the death of foetus. (Dellepiane 1959)

Pundal expressed the same view by stating the "abortion cell" (post partum type) with persistence of a majority of large parabasal cells for longer than 4 days indicated death of the foetus.In such cases, hormone treatment had no therapeutic role.

Ramos (1959) considered the utilization of urinary sediment smear for the diagnostic cytology on account of the passage of blood in cases of threatened abortion. He found that nearly 20 – 60% parabasal cells were present in the urocytogram in the abortion cases, a sign of combined oestrogen – progesterone deficiency.

Langreder and Merker (1954) were unable to find abortion cells (postpartum) in the urocytogram of abortion cases.

Later Meyer and Von Haam (unpublished data 1961) examined 100 catheterized specimens of urine, one specimen from each pregnant women, with the clinical diagnosis of incomplete abortion and using non pregnant women as control. He used the Millipore filter technic for preparation of the urinary sediment smears. They could find characteristic postpartum cells in 25% of the smears of pregnant patients with threatened abortion and 5% non pregnant cases. Perhaps one may say that persistent presence of postpartum cells is the best proof of foetal death in the pregnant cases. The abortion cell is small, rich in glycogen, resembling the postpartum cells, which in abortion cases is labeled as "abortion cell". Papanicolaou depicted in his atlas "two cells" which he was tempted to call the abortion cells. These were acidophilic, navicular shaped cells with a pyknotic nucleus.

d. **Incomplete Abortion:** Fletcher (1940) suggested the vaginal smear as a means of recognizing incomplete abortion in women whose vaginal bleeding was of undetermined significance. He believed the appearance of basal layer cells in association with many phagocytes to be diagnostic of an incomplete abortion.

In most of the cases, syncitiotrophoblast, endometrial cells, red blood cells, leucocytes and some endocervical cells with products of conception in addition to changed hormonal pattern are found in vaginal smears of incomplete abortion. Although the features of inevitable and incomplete abortions are identical, but syncitiotrophblasts are rarely seen in the incomplete abortion, which differentiates it from the inevitable abortion.

e. **Missed Abortion:** When the cases of moderate cornification in threatened abortion were treated with stilboestrol, instead of returning to the normal pregnancy smear there was an increase in cornification index, although the symptoms of threatened abortion had disappeared. These cases of missed abortion eventually clinically manifested. The early smears demonstrated signs of termination of pregnancy; and such confirmation on smear, thus obviates days and weeks of false hope,leading to expensive treatment regimen, which was certainly a futile prenatal prolongation of an inevitable outcome. (Birtch-1961).

f. **HabitualAbortion:** The relationship of the foetus and the placenta in a pregnant woman can be regarded as that of a homograft, at least to the extent that it involves the paternal fraction (Thomas et al 1959 and Bardawil et al 1962). The Pregnant women with the a history of foetal loss in cases of abortion showed a high

In menopausal women of similar age group, the percentage of KPI was low, while parabasal cells were higher in the vagina as compared to that in the labia minora. This wide difference of parabasal cells indicated that atrophy of upper part of a vagina may be more profound than in the labia minora for the same degree of estrogen deficiency.

B.MENOPAUSE AND ITS RELATION WITH MALIGNANCY OF THE FEMALE GENITAL TRACT

Catherine et al (1974) performed a short oestrogen test, in women forty years of age or older, as an aid to the differential diagnosis in those who exhibited evidence of epithelial atrophy with equivocal cellular criteria in their vaginal smears.

The authors published the work following their experience of administering the modified oestrogen test to a large number of women for a period of over 20 years, to learn the specificity and sensitivity in the detection of atypia in patient, who had post menopausal atrophic changes.

A total of 48654 patients who were 40 years of age or over were reviewed, of which 9897 patients exhibited atrophic changes of the vaginal epithelium. A total of 598 cases were selected for the oestrogen test (that is, 6.04%) among those who revealed atrophic cell changes (or 1.28% of all women forty years of age or older). The Modified Oestrogen test: One of these was administered to each patient

1. Oral administration of 1 mg of diethyl-stilbesterol daily through five days with repeat smears two days after the cessation of test therapy

2. Oral administration of 3.75 mgm conjugated oestrogen (Premarin) daily in divided dosages through five days with repeat smear two days after the completion of therapy.

3. Intramuscular injection of 20 mg long acting oestrogenic substance with repeat smear (vaginal) seven days after the test.

4. Local administration 0.5 mg diethyl stilbestrol for 3 days (vaginal suppositories) with repeat smear on the fifth day.

In this study, 96% women selected the oral administration test (no.1). oestrogen

Among these 598 patients with equivocal atrophic vaginal smears, who underwent the oestrogen test, the repeat smear revealed 11 carcinoma in situ, 26 invasive epidermoid carcinoma and in 31 cases malignancies other than a squamous cell carcinoma. Of the 598 cases, 231 (that is, 38.6%) cases required a repeat smear within 120 days and another 133 (that is, 22.2%) cases, within 210 days. The rest of the cases were lost to follow-up and had no repeat smears.

Following the short term administration of the oestrogen test in women with epithelial atrophy, the following changes were observed as a response to the test dose:

1. The background became clean in the vaginal smears.

2. Superficial and intermediate cells became the predominant cell types in the vaginal smears on account of maturity of all the layers of the squamous epithelium.

3. Free nuclei and degenerative cell changes were diminished.

4. Squamous metaplasia increased especially in the endocervical and also in the ecto-cervical cells.

5. Previously present parabasal cells disappeared or reduced in number after oestrogen test.

6. There was an apparent "hormonal deafness" of malignant tumour cells to the administration of sex steroid as described by Boschann(Personal Communication). Thus if the malignant tumour cells were present, the repeat smears showed clear evidence of malignant cells among the abundant mature squamous cells.

diabetes, heart and circulatory diseases, cirrhosis of the liver, renal diseases, central nervous system disorders and with Digitalis therapy. The KPI, MI and MV indices served as good indicators of oestrogen activity. The results of the above were as follows:

1. No rise in oestrogen activity in the vaginal epithelium of diabetics who were on therapy and diet control.

   On the other hand Magie (1967) reported that in women with atleastone year of menopause, aged 44 years to 80 years who were clinically diabetic, (with impaired glucose tolerance test), there was increased oestrogen level in the vaginal smears of two third of patients. The endometrial biopsy of these cases revealed glandular hyperplasia and endometrial carcinoma in one third cases as a result of high levels of oestrogenfor a prolonged period. In these cases, the sequence of impaired carbohydrate metabolism leads to excess oestrogen production which is responsible for the endometrial pathology.

2. In cirrhosis of the liver, there was no evidence of increased oestrogen,although it has been generally believed that the conjugation of oestrogen is impaired in this disease leading to an increase in the level of the oestrogen hormone

3. In rural patients with similar diseases, lower values were observed, but since the number of cases were few, a confirmation of this was not possible.

4. Patients with cardiovascular and central nervous system disease, arthritis, cases with fractures, none of them showed any abnormal level of oestrogen activity.

5. Patients on digitalis therapy exhibited increased oestrogen like effect confirming the report of other investigators (Brunori 1965, Charles 1966 and Navab et al 1965). This reaction is explained by the similarity in the molecular structure of the active principle of digitals glycoside (glucose) and that of oestrone. On the contrary Gorden et al found no increase in maturation values in their study (1966) in digitalis therapy patients.

6. The incidence of vaginitis was high in postmenopausal women but a marked decrease was found in digitalis therapy cases.

The relatively low incidence of atrophy and the finding of an adequate maturation of the vaginal epithelium in the majority of cases, reported by all the workers in this field, indicates that oestrogen treatment in menopausal women should not be used indiscriminately. An accurate cytohormonal evaluation should always be carried out before and after treatment for the assessment of the effect of therapy.

Investigations of Papaniculaou (1933) to date and the reports of large numbers of workers in this field have proved the value of vaginal cytology in the assessment of endocrine activity. Papanicolaou in 1945, while working on detection of cancer cells in the urinary sediment smears discovered that significant cytologic changes could be noted much more readily in these than in the vaginal smears. Thus his attention was diverted to the study of urinary sediment smears (catheterised specimens) in pregnant females (1947). He found that this simple rapid cytologic technique can easily be utilised in pregnancy, as morphologically cells show great similarity with that of the vaginal cells.

Later Del-Castillo et al (1948-49) also described that urinary sediment smears show similar variations of hormonal activity as in vaginal smears and subsequent studies of Lencioni 1963–69 demonstrated the usefulness of this technique in hormonal cytology.

In 1965–66 Delcastillo et al discovered a similar cycle in the cells exfoliated from the inner surface of labia minora in child bearing age and prepubertal girls. He performed this investigation also in menopausal and pregnant women and proved that labia minora smear (nymphocytogram) was equally an accurate index of ovarian activity.

reliable technique for the prediction of pregnancy outcome. It is imperative to determine whether or not treatment is necessary (in each case) :treatment based solely on history of recurrent abortion willprove to be expensive as well as inconvenient tothe patient.

MacRae (1967) while working on the correlation of vaginal cytology and hormonal assays in Pregnancy stated that" as a general rule, there is a good correlation between the vaginal cytology and urinary hormone output in normal pregnancy, while some complications of pregnancy do not show this relationship. Some cases of threatened abortion, and especially in cases of recurrent abortions, poor progesterone effect and high karyopyknotic indices (abnormal pregnancy smears) with normal levels of urinary hormones were observed. When the target cell shows complete or incomplete response to exogenous hormone, it is suggestive of either of these:

a. failure of enzyme formation at the cell membrane.

b. enzyme block

In such cases, enzyme treatment is prescribed. MacRae again attempts to emphasize that response of the cell is a rather truer guide to hormone action than the hormonal assays.

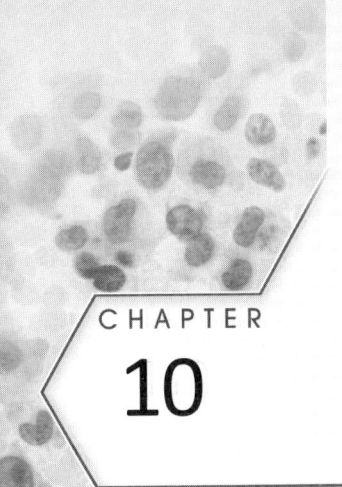

Correlation of Cytohormonal and Cytoenzyme Activity in Vaginal Epithelium in Women with Abortions

Dudkiewicz in 1977 published his work on the correlation between the cytohormonal indices and cytoenzyme activity of the exponents of Oestrogen and Progesterone occurring in the vaginal epithelium in both normal pregnancies and threatened abortion.

Cytohormonal exponents of oestrogen and progesterone activity in the vaginal epithelium recognize the dependence of the activity and quantity of certain enzymes upon similarsex hormones. A large number of workers including Atkinson and Engle (1947), Ayre (1951), Matter (1955), Barbour(1961), Jonek and Steplewski (1963, 1964), Tichy et al (1964), Toth et al (1966),and Cieciura et al (1970) have already shown a correlation between the activity of the three enzymes Alkaline phosphatase, Adenosine Tri Phosphatase, $NADH_2$ t.r. and the levels of the hormone oestrogen. A similar correlation between the intensity of cytochemical reactions for the two constituents Acid phosphatase, Glycogen with the quantity of Progesterone has been experimentally demonstrated by Atkinson and Engle (1947), Barbour (1961), and Toth and Gimes(1966).

Initially the science of vaginal exfoliative cytology as the marker of sex hormone activity, was applied in the evaluation of placental function disturbances; later Dudkiewicz in 1977 demonstrated a positive correlation between the cytohormonal indices

and cytoenzymatic activity of oestrogen and progesterone in the vaginal epithelium of normal pregnancies as well as a large number of threatened abortion cases. The results were as follows:

a. Correlation between the cytochemical reactions for alk-phosphatase (ALP.), ATPase, $NADH_2$t.r. and oestrogen activity in the vaginal epithelium was represented as the cytohormonal indices EI, KPI.

b. Correlation between the intensity of cytochemical reactions of enzymes Acid Phosphatase (ACP), Glycogen (as PAS reaction) with progesterone activity in the vaginal epithelium was represented by the cytohormonal indices FCI, CCI.

The above study included 185 cases of Threatened Abortion and a control group of 5 pregnant women with normal gestation by the 12 th week:

– In cases of threatened abortion, the usual gestation age ranged between 7 – 16 weeks. The vaginal smears were stained by Shorr's technique:

– All cases of inflammatory smears were eliminated.

– The indices calculated in each case were KPI, EI, CCI, FCI.

– Cases were divided into four groups, based on the classification of Dudkiewicz 1968 and 1974. The most important cytologic criteria of this gradation was as follows:

In menopausal women of similar age group, the percentage of KPI was low, while parabasal cells were higher in the vagina as compared to that in the labia minora. This wide difference of parabasal cells indicated that atrophy of upper part of a vagina may be more profound than in the labia minora for the same degree of estrogen deficiency.

B.MENOPAUSE AND ITS RELATION WITH MALIGNANCY OF THE FEMALE GENITAL TRACT

Catherine et al (1974) performed a short oestrogen test, in women forty years of age or older, as an aid to the differential diagnosis in those who exhibited evidence of epithelial atrophy with equivocal cellular criteria in their vaginal smears.

The authors published the work following their experience of administering the modified oestrogen test to a large number of women for a period of over 20 years, to learn the specificity and sensitivity in the detection of atypia in patient, who had post menopausal atrophic changes.

A total of 48654 patients who were 40 years of age or over were reviewed, of which 9897 patients exhibited atrophic changes of the vaginal epithelium. A total of 598 cases were selected for the oestrogen test (that is, 6.04%) among those who revealed atrophic cell changes (or 1.28% of all women forty years of age or older). The Modified Oestrogen test: One of these was administered to each patient

1. Oral administration of 1 mg of diethyl-stilbesterol daily through five days with repeat smears two days after the cessation of test therapy

2. Oral administration of 3.75 mgm conjugated oestrogen (Premarin) daily in divided dosages through five days with repeat smear two days after the completion of therapy.

3. Intramuscular injection of 20 mg long acting oestrogenic substance with repeat smear (vaginal) seven days after the test.

4. Local administration 0.5 mg diethyl stil-bestrol for 3 days (vaginal suppositories) with repeat smear on the fifth day.

In this study, 96% women selected the oral administration test (no.1). oestrogen

Among these 598 patients with equivocal atrophic vaginal smears, who underwent the oestrogen test, the repeat smear revealed 11 carcinoma in situ, 26 invasive epidermoid carcinoma and in 31 cases malignancies other than a squamous cell carcinoma. Of the 598 cases, 231 (that is, 38.6%) cases required a repeat smear within 120 days and another 133 (that is, 22.2%) cases,within 210 days. The rest of the cases were lost to follow-up and had no repeat smears.

Following the short term administration of the oestrogen test in women with epithelial atrophy, the following changes were observed as a response to the test dose:

1. The background became clean in the vaginal smears.

2. Superficial and intermediate cells became the predominant cell types in the vaginal smears on account of maturity of all the layers of the squamous epithelium.

3. Free nuclei and degenerative cell changes were diminished.

4. Squamous metaplasia increased especially in the endocervical and also in the ecto-cervical cells.

5. Previously present parabasal cells disappeared or reduced in number after oestrogen test.

6. There was an apparent "hormonal deafness" of malignant tumour cells to the administration of sex steroid as described by Boschann(Personal Communication). Thus if the malignant tumour cells were present, the repeat smears showed clear evidence of malignant cells among the abundant mature squamous cells.

- **Type IV**

  Cytolysis +++: In these cases, statistically there was no significant difference in the reactions of the enzymes when compared to controls, except the reaction for PAS, which was more intense than in the controls. This group showed 16.7% abortion rate while 83.3% were successful pregnancies. Similar findings have been reported by Wisniowska (1970).

  It is observed that in a normal pregnancy, glycogen in the vaginal epithelium increases up to the 10th week of gestation and remains at that level up to the 18th week. The high level of glycogen results from the high levels of sex hormones secreted from the placenta. The intense cytochemical reaction observed in cytolytic cases is probably not associated with hormonal disturbances. The excessive cytolysis depends on the abundant growth of the Deoderlein bacilli. Zidovsky's opinion (1964) is that cytolysis in the vaginal pregnancy smears results from an intermediate glycogen rich layer inadequately covered by the superficial layer hence easily subject to destruction by the Deoderlein bacilli.

In threatened abortions, statistical analysis showed a positive correlation between the cytochemical exponents of oestrogen activity (ALP, ATP-ase, $NADH_2tr$) and cytohormonal indices (KPI and EI). Further a negative correlation between the PAS reaction for Glycogen and Acidphosphatase was observed with the cytohormonal activity (KPI and EI). While with greater increase in the intensity of PAS reaction for glycogen and ACP, there was a further decrease in EI and KPI. No correlation between the intensity of PAS reaction for glycogen and Alkaline phosphatase with the cytohomonal values FCI and CCI could be found. These findings are suggestive that cytologic smears like the cytochemical investigations give an insight into the placental function. On the basis of a distinct positive correlation between the cytochemical exponents of oestrogen activity (ALP, ATPase, $NADH_2t.r.$) and cytohormonal indices (KPI and EI), Dudkiewicz presumed that cytohormonal indices are of clinical value in cases of Threatened Abortions.

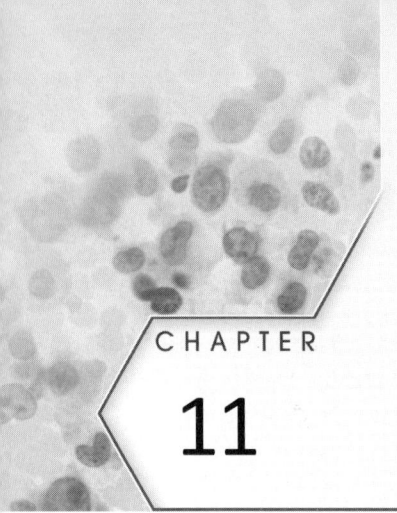

Cytohormonal Pattern in Late Abnormal Pregnancies and Associated Diseases

It is believed that vaginal cytology represents a useful tool for evaluating the course of pregnancy during the first trimester of pregnancy, but it has attracted a very little attention in the third trimester of pregnancy especially if associated with complications. Whereas contributions to the cytology of diabetes (Kamnitzer, 1959), and heart diseases (Leeton 1967) are scarce, those concerning the toxaemia of pregnancy are few (Misra,1969; Leeton,1967; Wood et al, 1961; Spira MacRac, 1960). The studies on the cytology of post-maturity are more extensive (Litchtfuss, 1959, Pundal, 1959, Dexeus et al 1966, Ohlenroth et al 1967, Palliez et al. 1968, Nunez et al 1968). On the other hand a large number of studies have been devoted to cytology at the end of the gestational period and to the controversy regarding its changing aspect by Pundal (1959), Lichtfus (1959), Abrams and Abrams (1962), Hindman et al (1962), Osmond-Clarke et al (1964), and Hammond et al (1965).

In obstetric practice miscellaneous tests have been developed to assess placental function test and the associated risk of perinatal death. These tests previously included the assessment of urinary excretion levels of oestradiol and pregnandiol, but-presently cytohormonal evaluation has been found to be the most sensitive, quick, economical and reliable method for assessment of placental functions. Both abortion and labour are known to be

associated with hormonal changes; similarly, changes that appear in the complications of pregnancy also have the same biological basis, that is, they are an expression of change in the "placental hormonal function".

Leeton (1967) analysed the placental function by studying the cytohormonal pattern, seven days prior to delivery and tried to predict the date of delivery and correlated the vaginal cytology to the outcome of the pregnancy. Most studies on placental function had been carried out on the basis of subjective criteria of cytology,whileLeeton tried to study the cytohormonal pattern in late abnormal high risk pregnancies, utilizing the six factors, some of which included certain objective criteria also for assessment. These were as follows:

1. Pregnancy–pattern _____ normal late pregnancy pattern
2. Navicular Cells _____ more than 25%
3. Karyopyknotic Index _____ less than 10%
4. Desquamation _____ marked
5. Rod like Nuclei _____ more than 20%
6. Red Blood Cells-or Mucous _____ Absent

The evaluation of smears was carried out on the basis of criteria used by Wood et al, (1961) and were graded as 1, 2, 3, as follows:

GRADING of Smears

Grade 1: Smears, which possessed all the six factors.

Grade 2: Smears, which presented at least four criteria

Grade 3: Smears, which possessed less than four criteria and persisted more than seven days.

Normal Pregnancy Smear: Normal Pregnancy 1,2,3 Smears were those that did not show progressive deterioration except the typical "at term" smear changes.

Abnormal Pregnancy Smears: When 1, 2, 3, smears showed either a progressive deterioration in grading or which possessed more than 5% parabasal cells.

The findings in hypertension and pre-eclampsia in Leeton's series closely corresponded to the results of Wood et al (1961).

The pregnancy cases showing grade 1 or 2 type of smears had a good prognosis and none of these were associated with anoxia of the foetus. There was no statistical difference in the occurrence of grade 1 or 2 found in normal pregnancy to that found in complicated cases except that of Rhesus isoimmunization.

The complicated cases with grade 3 vaginal smears revealed several episodes of clinical foetal anoxia which were noted after either amniotomy or on onset of labor. These cases carried a less favourable prognosis than grade 1 or 2 smears.

In patients with normal vaginal cytology, none of the babies were lost and intervention was not required at any stage of pregnancy. However in two cases, where abnormal smears were seen, foetal death followed a few days after obtaining the smears. The patients who delivered normal healthy babies, did not reveal abnormal cytology at any stage. In relation to the development of foetal anoxia and subsequent foetal death, it would appear that the abnormal vaginal smear carried a very grave prognosis as foetal death was imminent within a few days.

The above results indicate that vaginal cytology is a true guide for an obstetrician especially in the management of the frequent dilemma of prolonged pregnancies and their management. The pregnancies with grade 1 and 2 smears did not require any medical intervention, while induction of labour needed only to be carried out in those pregnancies with grade 3, and caesarean section could be preferred in those patients with abnormal vaginal smears in order to avoid foetal anoxia. In such cases, as anoxia always occurs after induction or spontaneous labour.

A contemporary worker MacRae (1967) stated that there is a close relationship between vaginal cytology and hormone assays. Although in normally progressing pregnancies there is a close harmony between the colpocytogram and urinary hormone excretion, dissociation between the two was found in certain cases of abnormal pregnancy. It is said that once progesterone predominance is established, then vaginal cytology may not reflect the hormonal variation in cases of recurrent abortions and chronic hypertension. It was noted that a fall in oestrogen levels in these cases was associated with a normal pregnancy smear, therefore he concluded that cytology did not have any prognostic value in these complications.

Another contemporary worker Malek et al (1967) carried out a study where he assessed multiple factors, using the cytohormonal study as an index in determining the biological mechanism that initiates spontaneous labour at "at term"; "premature and early rupture of foetal membranes", and in "pregnancy with delayed term". The cytologic evaluation provided an estimate of the quality of the hormonal preparation for labour. In this way, vaginal cytology could guide the clinician when the preparation for labour was distinct (perfect) and when it was imperfect, thus assisting them in making the decision on when to induce or enhance uterine contractions or when to perform caesarean section to save the precious child.

Labour is associated with hormonal changes, it is also believed that the changes which appear in complicated pregnancies also have the same biological basis, that is, they are an expression of the change in the "placental hormonal function". Hormonal production of the placenta is said to be a secondary manifestation of the metabolic activities of the placenta, therefore Nyklicek (1968) carried out multiple laboratory procedures–urocytogram, vaginal wall biopsy, serum assessment of Alkaline Phosphatase, plasma protein (by electrophoresis) of the mother and the new born child as a complement to vaginal cytology. All the tests were performed on the day of delivery. In this study, the purpose of assessment of urocytology and histopathology was to evaluate the hormonal function of the placenta, while biochemical estimations were done to ascertain the metabolic function of the placenta. Nyklicek found colposcopy to be the most sensitive, easy, quick and reliable procedure and a well established tool to assess the placental function when compared to other laboratory investigations.

Nyklicek (1972) added the technique of Amnioscopy as a complement to vaginal cytology along with hormonal assay of estriol in the urine. Amnioscopy when compared with the result of vaginal hormonal cytology in cases of prolonged pregnancy (regressive smears) showed green colouration of amniotic fluid (meconium of the foetus) in two cases. This indicated foetal anoxia,requiring immediate induction of labour. Thus the vaginal cytology has been used as a method of follow up of hormonal function of placenta and amniosocopy as a procedure diagnosing acute danger of anoxia of the foetus.These methods were found complementary to each other.

Sen and Langley (1972) studied the vaginal cytology to assess the outcome of pregnancy in Threatened abortion, Habitual abortion pre-eclamptic toxaemia, essential hypertension, "small for date" babies and intrauterine death. Further a comparison of smear results was made with the predication of hormone assays.

Cytohormonal analysis was based on KPI, EI, bacterial flora and clumping. Five grades (grades A to E) of smears were described. This study revealed that vaginal cytology was a better diagnostic tool in threatened abortion as incidence of foetal loss bears a direct relationship to the grading of smears, as there were 83% Live births in grade A and 83% foetal loss in grade E.

There was a statistical significant correlation between the foetal loss and abnormal cytology in threatened abortion and habitual abortion, but not in pre-eclamptic toxaemia and other complications occurring in late pregnancies. Further it was noted that hormone assays were not a better prognostic index in early pregnancy than were the vaginal smears.

Bercovici et al. (1973) tried to evaluate the vaginal cytology in the third trimester of pregnancy with complications. Like Leeton he also was of the opinion that changes which normally occur at term and those we find in complications of pregnancy at the end of gestation, both depend on the hormonal function of placenta. Bercovici et al studied vaginal smears of 106 cases of "**at term**" pregnant women between 38 – 40 weeks of gestation and obtained at least two smears from the lateral vaginal wall in each case. The Leeton technique was used for smear preparation and the smears were stained using Papanicolaou method. Leeton and other European workers had used the Shorr's method for staining. The smears were evaluated by a more simple technique than Leeton. Bercovici et al (1973) utilized only two criteria for assessment of smears, that is, tendency to grouping, clustering or agglutination and karyopyknotic index (Table 11.1). These smears after evaluation and grouping were finally correlated with the outcome of delivery and Apgar score of the living new born child. The grouping of smear was as follows:

Table 11.1: Shows criteria of grouping

Group:	Type of Pregnancy Smear	Criteria	
		Cluster	KPI
Group 1:	Normal pregnancy smear	+++	<10%
Group 2:	Slight progesterone deficiency	++	5–15%
Group 3:	Marked progesterone deficiency	+ or 0	> 15%
Group 4:	Marked Progesterone with oestrogen Deficiency*—** Bercovici et al 1973	0	Less than 5%

*mostly Intermediate cells with moderate oestrogen deficiency
**mostly Parabasal cells in marked oestrogen deficiency, both have less than 5% K.PI

Group 1: The normal pregnancy group one corresponds to the pregnancy – prior to term of Lichtfus (1959), Pundal (1959) and Lemberg; Stamm-Watteville (1955), to the good pregnancy smear of Wood et al. (1961), to the third trimester pattern of Abram and Abram (1962), and to the late pregnancy smear of Zidovsky (1961).

Group 2: of slight progesterone deficiency corresponded to "pregnancy at term" of Lichtfus(1959), Pundal (1959), Lemberg, Stamm-Watteville (1955) and Zidovsky (1961).

Group 3: of marked progesterone deficiency corresponded to the "abnormal pregnancy smear of Wood et al (1961) and "clearly at term" smear of Zidovsky (1961) and "Superfizialzelltyp" of Ohlenroth and Severin (1967).

Group 4: of marked progesterone and oestrogen deficiency corresponded to "pregnancy regressive" type of Nyklicek 1959, to the postpartum of Lichtfus (1959), and Pundal (1959) and to the "regressive type" of Ohlenroth and Severin (1967).

Bercovici et al (1973) from the above observation revealed that 80% of the "at term" smears (out of 106) were of grade I characteristic of normal pregnancy and the rest (20%) showed features of mild progesterone deficiency. Only five out of 15 heart cases, two out of eight diabetic, two out of nine severe toxaemia and three out of 32 post maturity cases, all belonged to the mild progesterone deficiency (i.e. group II).

The marked deficiency type of smear (grade 3) was found in one mild to moderate toxaemia, in four of severe toxaemia and three of post maturity patients. Patients with marked deficiency of progesterone in their smears should be considered as having placental dysfunction and in consequence should be delivered immediately.

The rate of medical interventions performed in patients with normal pregnancy cytology smears was 33% and in those with hormonal deficiencies was 45%. The high medical intervention rate clearly demonstrates that vaginal cytology is a useful tool to evaluate placental function in complications of the third trimester of pregnancy.

Pundal (1959)who led cytology work in pregnancy patients; during the symposium on "hormonal cytology in pregnancy "stated that" if the vaginal smear presents changes in the placental function, these are only related to the regressive changes and these cannot be used to diagnose abnormal pregnancy or even to judge the seriousness of pregnancy complications.

Leeton (1967) also found some cases with persistent grade 3 smears with abnormal cytology in late abnormal pregnancy, four cases of postmaturity and four cases of antepartum haemorrhage, who were treated with Caesarean section or surgical induction, and thus saved the babies. Two cases with abnormal smear, one with hypertension at week 35 and one of near term, could not be salvaged. One patient of antepartum hemorrhage at 36 weeks with an abnormal smear delivered an asphyxiated baby on spontaneous delivery.

Zidovsky et al (1967) also indicated the importance of cytology in relation to foetal survival in toxaemia; pregnancy, Rh-sensitization and diabetes. They noted that any significant deviation in these cases from the normal hormonal pattern before 38 weeks was associated with an increased risk of foetal death, irrespective of the underlying disease. Similar findings had been also reported by Wood et al (1961) in cases of toxaemia and maternal hypertension. These views finally prove the finding of Pundal that regressive smears are the only helpful finding in vaginal cytology of late abnormal pregnancy.

Bercovici et al (1973) were able to find a high degree of correlation between the vaginal cytology smears and the Apgar score of the newborns. In 92% cases of "at term" patients with complications, who presented with smears of normal and slight progesterone deficiency effect (grade 1, 2) the neonate had a high Apgar score at birth. In the four patients presenting marked progesterone deficiency, two of the neonates were born with a low Apgar score and two with a medium Apgar score. On the other hand eight patients with normal pregnancy smears delivered babies with medium Apgar scores. This clearly indicates that Apgar score is also influenced by obstetric conditions at birth and type of delivery and may be diagnosed via the vaginal cytology.All workers in the field agreed in concluding that cytohormonal assay may represent a useful method for monitoring the placental function in the third trimester of pregnancy, particularly with regressive smears and when it is correlated with clinical data and other laboratory investigations.

In conclusion we can say that hormonal-cytology inspite of its limitations, is an easy diagnostic tool for abnormal pregnancy smears as well as it detects the foetal distress directing the clinical management in majority of the cases.

It is important to note that HPV is one of the most common sexually transmitted infections in 70 – 80% of sexually active female (Ault K.A. 2006).HPV may be a risk factor for "Preterm birth" and spontaneous abortion, and placental abnormalities may result from placental infections with HPV. (Gomez et al 2008 and Hermonant et al 1998).

In vitro studies have shown that HPV can infect the foetus via transplacental transmission (Sarkola et al 2008 and Rombaldi et al 2008). Cervical cytology is an effective tool for screening pregnant women for this infection and inflammation and predicting the pregnancy outcome (Zuo et al 2011).

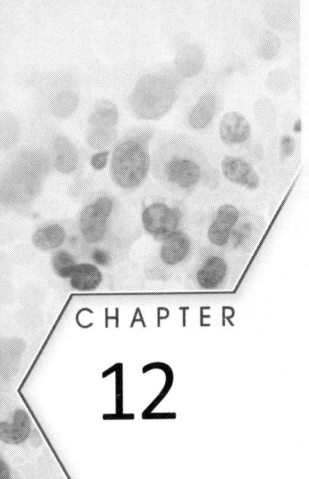

Cytohormonal Profiles of Amenorrhoea

According to endocrine cytology, the menstrual cycle depends on the interplay of hormones secreted by the "Hypothalamus – Pituitary – Ovarian Uterine Axis, (discussed in Chapter 2)."

Any functional or organic disorder of the above organs causes cessation of the normal menstrual cycle called "Amenorrhoea". The underlying causes can be:

1. **Physiological, eg. in Pregnancy, Lactation and Menopause.**
2. **Pathological, which is further divided into primary and secondary.**

Primary Amenorrhoea is one of the important symptoms of somatosexual disturbances (Syndromes) of different origins, which is mostly congenital, thus a wide spectrum of various cytologic patterns are observed.

Primary Amenorrhoea is defined as a somato-sexual disorder present before the age of puberty and the patient has never menstruated.

Secondary Amenorrhoea appears after puberty, as the acquired glandular lesion sets in. There is cessation of menstruation following the onset of the normal menstrual cycle at puberty. Secondary amenorrhoea can be temporary or permanent, depending on the nature of the disturbance.

The main difference between Primary and Secondary Amenorrhoea is that the time of onset is at variance. The final diagnosis of the syndrome, causing the amenorrhoea is not dependent only on hormonocytology. It requires a complete clinical, cytogenetic, morphological and cytohormonal profile of the patients. All investigations are required to be correlated with the cytologic pattern and the diagnosis possibly made with the help of the endocrinologist.

a. The classifications available in literature are three for Primary Amenorrhoea:

1. **By Dr Erica Wachtel (1966)**–based on the site of lesion (organ involved in the lesion).
2. **Ruiz and Teter (1968)**–mainly described cytohormonal profile and the distinction was made based on the origin of Amenorrhoea.
3. **Batrinos and Eustratiades (1972) – based on:**
   a. Clinical Findings,
   b. Histological Findings,
   c. Chromosomal Analysis, and
   d. Cytohormonal Assessment

The Classification by Batrinos and Eustratiades

Is believed to be the most suitable classification:

a. The **clinical diagnosis** was based on clinical signs formulated and used in the department of endocrinology (Athens Medical School, Greece). These patients were classified according to the clinical sign, that is, **absence or presence of breast development.**

b. **Histological findings as per the Ovarian biopsy examination.**

c. **Chromosomal Analysis:—Sex chromatin examination**

d. **Cytohormonal Assesment based on the study of the various cytological Indicies**
   At least 5 vaginal smears were taken from each patient aged between 15 to 18 years with an interval of 3 to 5 days.

The hormonal assessment was carried out by estimating the general pattern as well as the percentage of each type of cell (Batrinos 1968). This included the study of MI, KPI, EI and CCI and FCI. According to the cell types,the smear of each patient was classified into one of the following cell patterns:

1. The superficial cell type–at least 20% in the smear
2. This intermediate cell type–majority of cells are intermediate
3. The parabasal cell type–at least 20% in the smear

DETAILS OF BATRINOS AND EUSTRATIADES CLASSIFICATION

In this study, 12 distinct syndromes were divided into the following three groups (1,2,3), based on a correlation of visible clinical signs and smear patterns in 138 patients, aged 15 to 18 years, over a period of four years.

Group 1: Patients without Breast development. (90 out of 92 cases showed Atrophic smears and two smears were of the intermediate cell type).

Group 1 was further **classified into three sub groups (a, b, c).**

a. **Normal Stature:** Those patients with normal growth, height, and presence of an ovary with normal histology. These represented the greatest percentage of cases (76 = 55%)

Etiologically

   i. **Hypothalamo–Hypophyseal system defect with secondary ovaian failure**
   The gonadotrophins in the urine were absent therefore it was labeled as the **hypogonadotropic amenorrhoea** (18 cases) with HMG Test *positive and M.I.100/0/0

   ii. **Primary Ovarian failure-**Gonadotrophins in high quantity in the urine because of lack of Oestrogen Inhibition. This was labeled as **hypergonadotropic amenorrhoea** (20 cases) with HMG* negative (no response of the ovary)

   iii. Rest of the 38 cases, could not be classified in any of the above groups, although total gonadotrophin hormone was found to be normal in these cases

HMG*: Human Menopausal Gonadotrophin Test. In this Test, 150 Units of HMG in five daily doses were given and an assessment of the ovarian response was studied via vaginal cytology (Batrinos et al 1969).

b. **Medium Stature** (Muscular development and virilisation Congenital Adrenal Hyperplasia (one case)

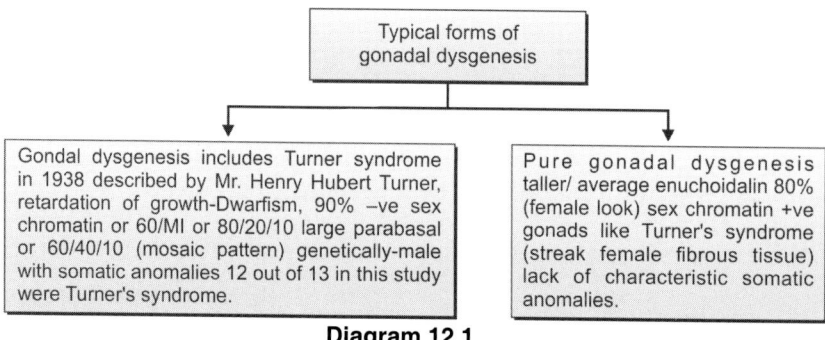

Diagram 12.1

c. **Short Stature:**It included the following groups

   i. Pituitary Dwarfism (two cases)

   ii. Typical forms of Gonadal Dysgenesis (diagram 12.1)

Group 2: Patients with Breast development (40 cases) In this group the hormono-cytological pattern* was as follows:

a. Parabasal cells in 13 cases (P)

b. Intermediate cells in15 cases (I)

c. Superficial cells in 12 cases (S)

*

P	I	S
13	15	12

Here the subgroups were classified basisthe condition of the uterus

a. **Those without palpable uterus (No uterus)**

   i. Testicular feminization (Mainly super-ficial cell types—(4 cases and 0:1:3*)

   ii. Syndrome of vaginal aplasia(No case)

b. **Those with atrophic uterus and ovarian hypofunction presented with breast development at puberty but did not menstruate. Gonadotrophins in the urine were found to be normal. (6 cases of ovarian hypofunction of undetermined origin and 4:2:0*)**

On account of Hypofunction of the Ovary, there were atrophic and intermediate cells in the vaginal smears.

c. **Normal or Atrophic Uterus:**

   i. Simple Pubertal retardation (12 cases and 5:2:5*)

   ii. Stein–Leventhal syndrome (six cases–confirmed **by ovarian biopsy, and 1:5:0*)**

   iii. Hypothalamic Disturbance,including Anorexia Nervosa (total four cases only, and 3:1:0*)

   iv. Destruction of the endometrium, mostly by Tuberculous Infection (eight cases, 0:4:4*)

Group 3: It comprises the Hermaphrodites, who may or may not have breast development

and were clinically distinguished by the intersexual development of External genitalia (six cases = 4.5%, and 5:1:0*)

The author studied a total of 138 cases, of which 108 showed Parabasal cells (78.3%), 18 Intermediate cells (13%) and13 superficial cells (8.7 %). The hormonocytological findings indicated the following pattern:

a. **Superficial cell pattern** belonged to the patients of the group with breast development, where there was a possibility of oestrogen secretion, such as simple pubertal retardation, endometrial infection and testicular feminisation.

b. **Parabasal cell type pattern** were suggestive of probable diagnosis of:

   i. Cases without breast development with an etiology where there is **complete absence** of ovarian function with MI as 100:0:0

   ii. Cases with breast development, showing MI 60:40:0; indicated ovarian **hypofunction.**

   Or

   iii. in the **Hermaphrodites**

c. Cases with Intermediate cell pattern:were observed in patients with various endocrinological conditions.

Conclusively these observations revealed that superficial cell smear type excludes the possibility of clinical syndrome belonging to the group without breast development, while the finding of a parabasal cell type smear orients the diagnosis towards this group.

Classification of Ruiz and Teter 1968

Ruiz and Teter (1968)reported that the primary amenorrhoea is related to the following syndromes.

1. **Gonadal Dysgenesis**

   a. It is mostly **Turner's Syndrome** with atrophic smear and M.I.80:20:0 or 60:40:0; and shows **large Parabasal cells** (Ruiz and Teter 1968).

b. A few pure gonadal dysgenesis cases show intermediate and superficial cells in the vaginal smears, M.I. 0:80:20, interpreted with respect to the other indicies as a moderate deficiency or slight oestrogen effect or an androgenic smear (Teter 1968). Most of these cases showed atrophic smear (Ruiz 1968).

2. a. **Pituitary Infantilism** with retardation of growth and **hypogonadotropic hypogonadism** with adrenal insufficiency due to severe hypothalamic lesion, show extremely **small parabasal cells** and M.I. 100:0:0.

 b. Various cytologic patterns fluctuating between Oestrogen Deficiency and slight oestrogen effect may occur in the syndrome of **premature Ovarian failure,** while some of the smears were also atrophic (Ruiz and Teter, 1968).

3. Ovarian Eunochoidism – shows atrophic patterns.

4. Testicular feminisation syndrome, can either have (a)superficial cells,or (b) intermediate cells.

5. Congenital Adrenal Hyperplasia – A variety of Smear Patterns are seen, that is, either completely atrophic or intermediate or androgenic.

 Thus, 80% of cells were atrophic and the remainder parabasal and intermediate (Ruiz L.1964).

6. Uterogenic primary amenorrhoea showed normal cytohormonal pattern

 Teter (1968) stresses that various syndromes in Primary Amenorrhoea showed a wide spectrum of cytologic patterns, therefore it was not possible to suggest a specific or typical pattern of hormonocytology in any of these cases. While Batrinos (1972) was of the opinion that lack of precision invalidates the vaginal cytology as an assay method for primary amenorrhoea, without the help of the clinician, and essentially the endocrinologist.

Even the other workers (Pundal 1957, Rakoff 1961, Watchtel 1966 and Wied 1964) in the field of endocrine cytology have mentioned that any information furnished by the vaginal cytology remains without any practical value unless it helps the clinician in making an accurate diagnosis.

Saraiya et al (1976) studied 300 cases of amenorrhoea, referred to the cytology clinic, Mumbai from Jan 1971 to June 1973. Out of 300 cases 60 were of primary amenorrhoea. They analysed the smears and correlated with the relevant clinical data and grouped these in 4 categories as suggested by Rakoff (1961).

The table No.12.1 shows smear pattern in primary amenorrhoea according to the age of the patients. Hormonal evaluation was possible in 41 cases out of 60 cases. 17 showed atrophic Smear Patterns, where as 34 cases revealed a various degree of epithelial proliferation (Prolif) and rest of the 19 cases were unsuitable for Cytohormonal analysis.

The authors found that in general it was difficult to study cytology in primary amenorrhoea especially in a very young and unmarried girls. Serial smears were contraindicated on account of risk of infection in these cases.

Table 12.1: Smear Pattern in Primary Amenorrhoea (Saraiya et al 1976)

Type	Age	No of Cases	Atrophic	Mild Prolif.	Good Prolif.	Progesterone	Unsuitable
Primary	<20–20–	36	16	18	2	—	10
60	35>35	24	1	10	3	1	9

b. **SECONDARY AMENORRHOEA:** Mills and Wilson (1969) carried out studies in 117 cases of Secondary Amenorrhoea, but diagnosis could finally be made in 105 cases relating all the patient's endocrine data.

In this group of 117 cases the age distribution was as follows:

a. 115 cases were of 17–30 years

b. 2 cases – one was 45 and the other was 46 years old

The results were as follow:

1. Polycystic Ovarian disease accounted for 50% of the cases of Mills and Wilson. The diagnosis in the Mills and Wilson cases was confirmed after studying the tissue removed on wedge resection of ovary, following which 16 of the women started-regular menstruation and six of the women went on to become pregnant.

2. The next most frequent diagnosis was that of Anorexia Nervosa, accounting for 17% of the cases. Restoration of normal weight brought about a return of menstruation in eight of the cases. These eight cases were treated with clomiphene therapy, four of the women became pregnant.

3. Among the rest of the cases, the diagnosis was as follows.

   a. Low BMR _____ seven cases.

   b. Psychological disorder _____ six cases.

   c. Two Cases each of–Obesity Amenorrhoea and Pituitary Tumour; three cases each of Ovarian Hypoplasia and Early Menopause

   d. one case each of (1) Hypopituitarism, (2) Cushing Syndrome, (3) Thyrotoxicosis, (4) Chromosomal mosaicism, xo/xy

Ferriman and Purdie (1965) have reported 70% cases suffering from polycystic ovarian disease among the 467 patients of Secondary Amenorrhoea. Hirsutes and post-pill amenorrhoea were strong pointers to such diagnosis. While anorexia nervosa and ovarian dysgenesis were found among the non-hirsute amenorrheic patients. No cytological findings were discussed in the cases of Mills and Wilson as well as Ferriman and Purdie.

Willis and Harley (1966), defined the vaginal smear pattern in certain cases of amenorrhoea as shown in Table 12.2; smears were collected from the lateral vaginal wall and stained by Shorr's stain

1. Hypertrophic-High oestrogen secretion—(40% KPI or more)

2. Eutrophic—Normal oestrogen secretion-level peaks in the middle of menstrual cycle and then falls.

3. Hypertrophic- Persistently high level of oestrogen which is of 3 types (a, b, c)

   a. Mild to Moderate: reveals fluctuations in KPI and EI

   b. Marked–KPI always remains low, that is below 10 %

   c. Very marked absolutelyintermediate cells or occasionally with KPI 2–3%.

4. **Atrophic:** Complete lack of oestrogen, shows complete absence of superficial eosinophilic and karypyknotic cells with occasional intermediate cells.

Note: In a case report of genetic cause of primary amenorrhoea, Anupama et al (2011) has reported that the proximal "p" as well as "q" arm deletions of X-Chromosome was found with severe type of abnormalities, resulting in Primary amenorrhoea. In a case of distal long "q" arm deletion of X- Chromosome, menarche may occur, followed by normal menstrual cycle, but fertility complications are reported.

Table 12.2: Vaginal Smear Patterns Associated with Amenorrhoea

Causes of amenorrhoea	Hyper-trophic	Eutrophic	*Hypotrophic* Mild to Moderate	Marked	Very Marked	Atrophic	Total Number of Patients
Disordered Cortico Hypothalamic function	–	14	21	2	1	0	38
Polycystic Ovary Syndrome	–	–	3	3	19	3	28
Ovarian Hyperfunction	13	–	–	-	–	–	13
Obesity	–	3	5	-	3	–	11
RRPituitary Insufficiency	–	–	–	4	3	–	7
Gonadal Dysgenesis	–	–	–	–	–	5	5
Hypothy-roidism	–	–	5	–	–	–	5
Total	13	17	34	9	26	8	107

CYTOHORMONAL ANALYSIS OF THE CLASSICIFICATION OF AMENORRHOEA BY DR. ERICA WATCHTEL

Dr. Erica Watchtel combined primary and secondary amenorrhoea and classified it according to organ wise lesions.

I have attempted to classify all lesions, described organwise, into groups of probable cytohormonal findings, observed by her and other workers.

1. Atrophic Smear:
   a. **Primary Pituitary Failure:**
   There is low FSH in these cases. It leads to secondary ovarian failure.
   Causes–Tumours of Pituitary– Adenoma, other lesions-Tuberculoma, Syphilitic lesion, vascular lesion–Simmond's disease or Frohlich's disease.
   b. **Primary Ovarian Failure:**
   FSH is high
   Gonadal Dysgenesis, (congenital)

Turner's Syndrome described by Henry Hubert Turner (1938). These cases are genetically male – sex chromatin negative - with often a Mosaic Pattern MI – 100:0:0. Hypogonadism,which is responsible for dwarfism in 90 % cases shows negative sex chromatin.

Acquired: Post-Operative,Inflammation (Tuberculosis, Syphilis, Mumps)or Radiation effect on ovary

2. **Cyclical Changes:** Uterine Disorders
   a. Congenital absence of Uterus or Hypoplasia and sex chromation positive
   b. Acquired Endometrial Lesions: Tuberculosis, Hysterectomy, very deep Curettage
   c. Non-functioning Endometrium (due to repeated curettage)

3. **High Proliferation Smear: (Persistent)**
   a. Oestrogen Producing Tumour–Thecoma, Granulosa Cell Tumour or Carcinoma (sex chromatin positive.)

b. Oestrogen producing Cyst – Sex Chromatin positive Follicular Cyst

c. Testicular feminization – Sex Chromatin Negative

4. Moderate Proliferation

a. Stein Leventhal Syndrome
Ovary is palpable and enlarged

b. Milder type psychogenic disorders with associated emotional factors

5. Secretory Pattern:

a. Persistent Luteal Cyst

b. Pseudocyesis (in both these cases, the pregnancy test is negative)

6. Intermediate Cell Proliferarion

a. MI – 0:80:20 – Pure gonadal Dysgenesis

b. Androgen producing Tumours and Adrenal hyperplasia

Androgen effect or mild oestrogenic effect is seen on Cytology or (b)Multi – Hormonal Effect may be seen.

Diagnosis is difficult in cases of Primary amenorrhoea on the basis of endocrine cytology, therefore the authors who classified amenorrhoea resulting from various syndromes have advised a consultation with the endocrinologist. Saraiya et al (1976) studied 300 cases of amenorrhoea out of which 60 cases were of primary amenorrhoea and 240 cases were of secondary amenorrhoea. The 240 cases were of further categorized into 4 groups according to Rakoff (1961). Cytohormonal analyses was carried out in 180 cases (Table 12.3) according to the age of the patients. Smear pattern in secondary Amenorrhoea Saraiya et al 1976.

Table 12.3:

Age Cases	No. of	Atro-phic	Mild Prolif.	Good Prolif	Proges-terone	Unsuit-Able
<20	4	1	11	4	2	6
20–30	185	15	76	33	20	41
>35	31	2	13	1	2	13
–	240	18	100	38	24	58

Dr.Saraiya's opinion is that exfoliative Cytology has a definite place in the diagnosis and management of amenorrhoea besides that it is the simplest and least expensive tool.

Details of smears pattern in the 4 categories as described by Dr. Saraiya were as follows.

1. Atrophic Smears: cellular pattern in 18 cases (10%) consisted of mainly parabasal cells, with a few intermediate cells. The EI and K.P.I were less than 10. The background consisted of several WBC's.There were absence of Cytolysis and Deoderlein bacilli were few.

This smear pattern indicates that ovarian function is absent or negligible. In these cases it was important to find out whether ovarian failure is primary or secondary to pituitary, which could be done by studying the response on administration of F.S.H (Follicle Stimulating Hormone). If no response than ovaries are permanently damaged. F.S.H is high in primary ovarian failure and low in secondary ovarian failure. The authors were not able to carry out this test.

Batrinos and Eutratiades (1972) carried out HMG (Human Menopausal Gonadotrophin) test to find out whether atrophy is due to primary or secondary ovarian failure in such cases.

According to Dr. Saraiya et al atrophic smear are observed in postpartum amenorrhoea or when ovaries are damaged by irradiation or severe infection for, e.g. Tuberculosis and premature menopause. Analysis of 18 cases was as follows.

- Postpartum amenorrhoea—one
- Normal size of uterus—6 out of these 15 cases 7 were fertile 8 infertile
- Smaller size of the uterus—9
- Premature menopause in 2 cases (Age above 35)

2. Smears of Mild Proliferation:- 100 cases (55%) predominant cellular pattern was of intermediate cells and there were a few superficial and a few parabasal cells. EI and

KPI varied between 10–30%. Cells were either single or in small groups. WBCS were present, but Cytolysis was absent and Deoderlein bacilli were few. This was the largest group in their study. In these cases serial smears were of great significance as ovarian function wax and vane. Among this group large number of cases were found to be suffering from pulmonary tuberculosis.

3. **Smears of good Proliferation-**38 cases (21%): Cellular Pattern was of intermediate cells. E.I and KPI were above 30%. Background appeared clean with absence of WBCS, Cytolysis and Deoderlein bacilli. There is persistent follicular phase. The response to ovulation inducing drugs was good and treatment with cyclic progesterone was successful.

4. **Progestrone effect 24 cases (14%):-**The cellular pattern was of intermediate cells in large and small placards there was marked folding of cell margins, cytolysis, WBC and Deoderlein were more in the background, which indicated recent ovulation. There was a good co-relation between the hormonal cytology and oestrgen excretion.

Dr. Saraiya opined that exfolitive cytology is simple and least expensive and plays an important role in the amenorrhoea related to ovarian and pituitary failure. In other cases it does not play a significant role. The overall study of serial smears has to be evaluated together with clinical data. For this the Cytologist must be familiar with basic endocrinology and interplay of sex hormones in health and disease. She agrees to the sugession of Dr. Wied (1968) that the dual speciaisation in cytopathology and endocrinology is necessary for reliable cytohormonal evaluation in amenorrhoea.

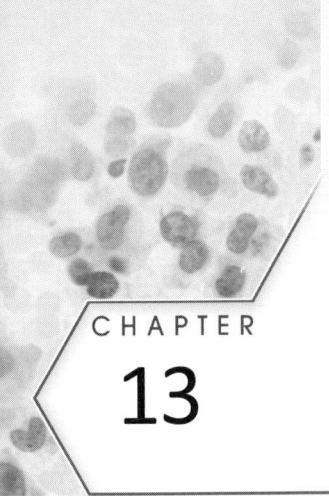

CHAPTER

13

Hormonal Cytology of Menopause Including Pre and Post Menopausal Phases

A. HORMONAL CYTOLOGY OF MENOPAUSE INCLUDING PRE AND POSTMENOPAUSAL PHASES

The premenopausal period varies from 41 to 50 years. It is a period of great physical symptomatic turbulence with gradual progressive alterations in the female hormonal status until menopause sets in. These changes are closely linked with the disturbances of hormonal balance and may manifest themselves clinically in the form of vasomotor instability producing symptoms such as hot flushes, palpitations, sweating, headaches and psychological illness for example, mood swings. The cytological changes in the smear patterns are variable and hence information will only be available by repeating smears at frequent intervals. Some women have, at first occasional and later increasingly frequent anovulatory cycles, characterised by irregular oestrogen production and absence of secretory changes. The features are reflected in the cytology as irregular karyopyknotic index curves and the absence of progesterone effect.

These are as follows (shown in Chapter 7)

i. Erratic Curve (Diagram 7.2A) Irregular menstrual cycle

ii. Hypo-Ovarian Curve (Diagram 7.2B) constantly low oestrogen level

iii. Inactive Curve (Diagram 7.2C) almost absence of oestrogen

iv. High Plateau Curve (Diagram 7.2D) Persistent high oestrogen level

It is observed that after castration or spontaneous menopause, the cytology goes through several phases:

The smears vary from highly proliferative to the atrophic type in the following phases.

a. Beginning,

b. Moderate,

c. Deep and atrophic.

The completely atrophic smears contain only immature parabasal cells with hyperchromatic nuclei, numerous leucocytes, RBC and necrotic debris. Occasionally a mixed type of smear, composed of superficial cells, parabasal cells is observed. After the cessation of ovulatory function it is reasonable to expect that smear becomes atrophic, however an atrophic smear is an exception rather than a rule.

The most common smear pattern in the few years following menopause is one of predominance of the intermediate cells with occasional superficial and parabasal cells. This intermediate cell type of smear is further classified by Pundal 1968 into two types.

a. Intermediate cells, having features same as seen in the normal menstrual cycle or in hypoestrogenic conditions. It is the only cell type which Pundal (1957) in his personal classification of menopausal

65

cytology called the "Intermediate Cell Type".

b. This smear consist of intermediate cells which are larger, single, and flat with hypochromatic cytoplasm and vesicular nucleus; and in this type, the leukocytes are rarely seen. This smear is identical with that observed when the cells are under the effect of testosterone in castrated women, called the "androgenic cell type". Its origin is proved by the complete hormonal assay of these cases by showing a predominance of 17 ketosteroids over oestrogen.

Biological Phases of Menopause: It is not possible to precisely fix the duration of the different cytologic phases but biologically one may distinguish two different phases of the post menopausal period (Pundal 1968)

1. The first phase is very long but with marked individual variation, and is called the residual postmenopausal phase. It is characterised by definitive arrest of the menstrual cycle, however there remains a certain hormonal activity, preventing the appearance of epithelial atrophy

2. The second phase which follows,is the phase of senility, during which the epithelial atrophy is usually completed. This distinction is helpful in the understanding of the various histologic and cytologic changes which appear in the vagina after the onset of menopause.

From the observations of Struthers (1956), it may be concluded that the cytologic changes associated with marked hormonal activity, in cases of surgical castration (or spontaneous menopause) cannot be the result of any ovarian activity. It is indicative of the interference of ovarian hormonal activity from another endocrine gland, that is, the adrenal cortex, as he observed that oophorectomy did not result in a higher incidence of atrophic smears. Further, many workers in this field (Meisels, Montalo Ruiz, Muth and Pundal) in the symposium on "Effects of endo-genous oestrogen" (1960),on the basis of their observations, suggested that the adrenal cortex could be responsible for the lasting oestrogenic activity till late in the postmenopausal phase. Therefore there maybe a phase, that is, the adreno-cortical phase between the cessation of ovarian activity and senility with complete epithelial atrophy.

Dr. Saraiya in the preliminary report (1969) has discussed hormonal cytology of menopause as the result of natural cessation of ovulation and after castration. The vaginal smear of natural menopause shows an oestrogen active epithelium and is characterized by superficial and intermediate cells MI 0/50/50. The cells lie discretely and the background is clean, as the time goes by regressive changes in the ovary occurs and MI shows a shift towards the left.

The cytology of castration is affected by either surgery or irradiation. The biological phases, observed were identical to other workers, as follows:

1. Beginning
2. Moderate
3. Deep and atrophic

In this surgical castration if hysterectomy with bilateral oophrectomy is performed, it is the experience of most of the workers that smears become atrophic very soon, that is within 4 to 6 weeks as a result of sudden withdrawl of oestrogen. The smear pattern passes very rapidly from the beginning to that of atrophy.

When castration is carried out by irradiation, it may be difficult to interpret SMEARS because of radiation changes, therefore these vaginal smears cannot be considered for pure hormonal evaluation.

An acceptable classification was agreed upon during the "Symposium on hormonal cytology" (1968), taking into consideration all these different hormonal activities and their cytologic reactions to represent a precise

hormonal cytodiagnosis, as far as the complexity of these particular hormonal activities can allow of such a differential diagnosis.

The classification described in the "Symposium on Hormonal Cytology" by Pundal 1968 is as follows:

1. **Smear of Superficial cell types**

   a. **MIa:** Mostly flat or slightly folded cells but without clusters.

   b. **MIb:** Mostly folded but single cells.

   c. **MIc:** Folded cells in clusters.

2. **Smears of Intermediate cell type**

   a. **MII:** The usual, intermediate of type of cells, which are the predominant elements of the smear. Parabasal cells are absent.

3. Smears of the parabasal or sub atrophic type

   a. **M III:** Intermediate and parabasal cells.

4. **Smears of the completely atrophic type (MVI)**

5. **The androgenic smear type (MA)**

6. **The cytolytic smear type (MC)**

7. **Mixed smear types**

   This classification is schematic, based mainly upon the predominant cell type except for some particular cell changes independent of the cell type. It usually permits hormonal analysis with the exception of majority of cases with mixed smears (Complex Adreno–Cortical Activity).

   For the menopausal women, cytohormonal norms were suggested by Meisels (1966) and Stone et al (1967). The cytohormonal readings by Meisels were based on the differential count of vaginal part of VCE (Vaginal Cervical Endocervical on a single slide) smears, stained by Papanicolaou method. This differential count included 5 types of squamous cells, assigned a specific value, which is as follows:

   i. Superficial Eosinophilic Cell – 1.0

   ii. Superficial Cyanophilic Cell – 0.8

   iii. Large Intermediate Cell – 0.6

   iv. Small Intermediate Cell – 0.5

   v. Parabasal Cell –0.0

   Percentage of each cell was multiplied by its value and the results added. The sum (without decimal) were called as **Oestrogenic Value**.

   The oestrogenic value, calculated on the basis of differential count was later labelled as Maturation value (MV) of Frost. Meisels in 1967, suggested to reduce the number of cell types to three, with little change in the value, as described by Frost in the Terminology symposium (1958).

   The change was as follows (1) Superficial Eosinophilic Pyknotic Cell = 1.0, Intermediate = 0.5, and Basal Cell = 0.0.

   The advantage of the Oestrogenic Value is that like MV it could easily be submitted for statistical analysis.

   Meisels in 1966 published a report on cytohormonal evaluation of 5920 menopausal women who could fulfil the following additional criteria:

a. Adequate clinical information regarding the age, date of last menstrual period, Pelvic Surgery or radiotherapy (if given)

b. Technically a good smear (after taking precautions)

c. No marked inflammatory changes with impaired morphology of vaginal cells were observed of Trichomonas Vaginalis infection or Moniliasis.

d. No hormonal treatment was given three months prior to the collection of smears.

The observations of the studies of Meisels (1966) revealed that:

1. The age distribution indicated a normal pattern between the ages of 45 to 64 years in 70% of the cases, and there was a variation in the age of onset of menopause.

2. It was found that mean oestrogenic values were quite comparable with age and time elapsed since menopause.

In this study of 5920 cases,Meisels found that an appreciable number of patients retain a cytologically detectable oestrogenic activity far into old age. He determined the hormone value range during menopause and established the criteria for selecting menopausal patients eligible for hormonal treatment on basis of the oestrogenic values. He found three levels of oestrogenic activity in the menopause, which were as follows:-

a. Absent or Very Low – (EV 0 – 49) Decreasing in value gradually, in about half of the patients, with increasing years of menopause. In 21% of the cases, complete atrophy (EV 0) was observed.

b. Moderate Value – (EV 50 - 64) was found in 40% cases, who maintained it throughout life.

c. High Value – (EV 65–Over) 10% cases only, who carried it far into the old age.

These results confirm the work of others, who reported persistent oestrogenic activity in the menopausal period (Struthers – 1956, Allende 1950, Masukawa, 1960, Ruiz 1964, Muth 1960, Peters, 1960).

In 1956, Struthers could find only 20.1% of atrophic smears in the group of 353 menopausal patients, which is almost exactly the same finding as observed later by Meisels in 1966. He further observed that even after 25 years of menopause, atrophic smears did not exceed 40%.

Later Joshi, Saraiya and Fernandes (1971) studied cytology in 475 cases of menopause, attending the cytology clinic of Cama and Albless Hospital, Mumbai from December 1969 to Ju;ly 1971. Among these inflammatory 52.6% and abnormal 12.14% smears were found. Cytohormonal evaluation was possible in 110 cases out of 429 with natural menopause. Out of these 429 cases50.9% showed considerable oestrogenic activity and maturity, which is comparable to the finding of the other worker. It was observed that there was a gradual decline of oestrgenic activity in the vaginal smears with the increasing duration of the menopause, further they

found that urocytogram was not suitable for hormonal study in these cases. As far as estimation of hormones was concerned, there was higher urinary oestrogen levels in the earlier years after the menopause and with more mature cells. They could estimate 24 hrs total urinary oestrogen in 52 cases according to the Brown flurometric method (1968). Abnormal smears were rare in asymptomatic and in cases with prolapsed of the uterus.

Stone et al (1967) also reported oestrogen like effect in the vaginal smears of 340 chronically ill postmenopausal women, aged 40 years to 98 years. The study of KPI, MI and MV was carried out in those women who were menopausal for at least two years. In this group, the longest period of menopause was 48 years. The smears were collected from the lateral wall of vagina and stained with standard Papanicolaou staining technique. Patients receiving oestrogen therapy, patients with malignancy and patients who failed to respond to vaginitis treatment were excluded from this study. Stone et al modified the oestrogenic value calculation that all the superficial cells (both oesinophilic and cyanophilic) were arbitrarily valued at 0.9. Therefore now the range of value (maximum) was MV–90, which could be compared with oestrogenic effect. The interpretation of MV requires to be matched with the age and patient history.

The results in healthy women showed that the predominance of low values (0–49) was 41% during first decade of menopause and as high as 82% in the 5th decade of menopause. The percentage of women with high maturation value (65–90) remained at approximately the same level, that is, 8.9% through the first 30 years of postmenopause, then dropped to 3% in the fourth decade and 0% in the fifth decade of menopause.

Stone et al (1967) carried out work in the chronically ill postmenopausal patients. The KPI, MI and MV indices were used in this study to correlate oestrogen like effect with

diabetes, heart and circulatory diseases, cirrhosis of the liver, renal diseases, central nervous system disorders and with Digitalis therapy. The KPI, MI and MV indices served as good indicators of oestrogen activity.The results of the above were as follows:

1. No rise in oestrogen activity in the vaginal epithelium of diabetics who were on therapy and diet control.

   On the other hand Magie (1967) reported that in women with atleastone year of menopause, aged 44 years to 80 years who were clinically diabetic, (with impaired glucose tolerance test), there was increased oestrogen level in the vaginal smears of two third of patients. The endometrial biopsy of these cases revealed glandular hyperplasia and endometrial carcinoma in one third cases as a result of high levels of oestrogenfor a prolonged period. In these cases, the sequence of impaired carbohydrate metabolism leads to excess oestrogen production which is responsible for the endometrial pathology.

2. In cirrhosis of the liver, there was no evidence of increased oestrogen,although it has been generally believed that the conjugation of oestrogen is impaired in this disease leading to an increase in the level of the oestrogen hormone.

3. In rural patients with similar diseases, lower values were observed, but since the number of cases were few, a confirmation of this was not possible.

4. Patients with cardiovascular and central nervous system disease, arthritis, cases with fractures, none of them showed any abnormal level of oestrogen activity.

5. Patients on digitalis therapy exhibited increased oestrogen like effect confirming the report of other investigators (Brunori 1965, Charles 1966 and Navab et al 1965). This reaction is explained by the similarity in the molecular structure of the active principle of digitals glycoside (glucose) and that of oestrone. On the contrary Gorden et al found no increase in maturation values in their study (1966) in digitalis therapy patients.

6. The incidence of vaginitis was high in postmenopausal women but a marked decrease was found in digitalis therapy cases.

The relatively low incidence of atrophy and the finding of an adequate maturation of the vaginal epithelium in the majority of cases, reported by all the workers in this field, indicates that oestrogen treatment in menopausal women should not be used indiscriminately. An accurate cytohormonal evaluation should always be carried out before and after treatment for the assessment of the effect of therapy.

Investigations of Papaniculaou (1933) to date and the reports of large numbers of workers in this field have proved the value of vaginal cytology in the assessment of endocrine activity. Papanicolaou in 1945, while working on detection of cancer cells in the urinary sediment smears discovered that significant cytologic changes could be noted much more readily in these than in the vaginal smears. Thus his attention was diverted to the study of urinary sediment smears (catheterised specimens) in pregnant females (1947). He found that this simple rapid cytologic technique can easily be utilised in pregnancy, as morphologically cells show great similarity with that of the vaginal cells.

Later Del-Castillo et al (1948-49) also described that urinary sediment smears show similar variations of hormonal activity as in vaginal smears and subsequent studies of Lencioni 1963–69 demonstrated the usefulness of this technique in hormonal cytology.

In 1965–66 Delcastillo et al discovered a similar cycle in the cells exfoliated from the inner surface of labia minora in child bearing age and prepubertal girls. He performed this investigation also in menopausal and pregnant women and proved that labia minora smear (nymphocytogram) was equally an accurate index of ovarian activity.

In menopausal women of similar age group, the percentage of KPI was low, while parabasal cells were higher in the vagina as compared to that in the labia minora. This wide difference of parabasal cells indicated that atrophy of upper part of a vagina may be more profound than in the labia minora for the same degree of estrogen deficiency.

B.MENOPAUSE AND ITS RELATION WITH MALIGNANCY OF THE FEMALE GENITAL TRACT

Catherine et al (1974) performed a short oestrogen test, in women forty years of age or older, as an aid to the differential diagnosis in those who exhibited evidence of epithelial atrophy with equivocal cellular criteria in their vaginal smears.

The authors published the work following their experience of administering the modified oestrogen test to a large number of women for a period of over 20 years, to learn the specificity and sensitivity in the detection of atypia in patient, who had post menopausal atrophic changes.

A total of 48654 patients who were 40 years of age or over were reviewed, of which 9897 patients exhibited atrophic changes of the vaginal epithelium. A total of 598 cases were selected for the oestrogen test (that is, 6.04%) among those who revealed atrophic cell changes (or 1.28% of all women forty years of age or older). The Modified Oestrogen test: One of these was administered to each patient

1. Oral administration of 1 mg of diethyl-stilbesterol daily through five days with repeat smears two days after the cessation of test therapy

2. Oral administration of 3.75 mgm conjugated oestrogen (Premarin) daily in divided dosages through five days with repeat smear two days after the completion of therapy.

3. Intramuscular injection of 20 mg long acting oestrogenic substance with repeat smear (vaginal) seven days after the test.

4. Local administration 0.5 mg diethyl stilbestrol for 3 days (vaginal suppositories) with repeat smear on the fifth day.

In this study, 96% women selected the oral administration test (no.1). oestrogen

Among these 598 patients with equivocal atrophic vaginal smears, who underwent the oestrogen test, the repeat smear revealed 11 carcinoma in situ, 26 invasive epidermoid carcinoma and in 31 cases malignancies other than a squamous cell carcinoma. Of the 598 cases, 231 (that is, 38.6%) cases required a repeat smear within 120 days and another 133 (that is, 22.2%) cases,within 210 days. The rest of the cases were lost to follow-up and had no repeat smears.

Following the short term administration of the oestrogen test in women with epithelial atrophy, the following changes were observed as a response to the test dose:

1. The background became clean in the vaginal smears.

2. Superficial and intermediate cells became the predominant cell types in the vaginal smears on account of maturity of all the layers of the squamous epithelium.

3. Free nuclei and degenerative cell changes were diminished.

4. Squamous metaplasia increased especially in the endocervical and also in the ecto-cervical cells.

5. Previously present parabasal cells disappeared or reduced in number after oestrogen test.

6. There was an apparent "hormonal deafness" of malignant tumour cells to the administration of sex steroid as described by Boschann(Personal Communication). Thus if the malignant tumour cells were present, the repeat smears showed clear evidence of malignant cells among the abundant mature squamous cells.

When conducting such a test, it is important to inform the pathologist that the sample is a repeat smear after the oestrogen test, since such samples require more intensive screening than do cell samples where the tumour diathesis may provide diagnostic clues.

This test is helpful in avoiding unnecessary biopsies in postmenopausal women, when an equivocal cell pattern is found to be unequivocally benign after the performance of an oestrogen test.

The oestrogen test is also helpful in detecting the presence of the squamous cell carcinoma or a dysplasia of uterine cervix as the malignant cells appear less degenerated in repeat smears. After cessation of the short term test, there was a gradual return to the atrophic cell pattern in most of these cases, as early as 15 days and as late as 10 months.

The Oestrogen test is not helpful in the diagnosis of the endometrial carcinoma.

Llusia (1977) reported that a considerable number of the menopausal women, who had proliferative vaginal smears, indicating a certain level of oestrogen production, showed no significant correlation with:

a. Age since menopause

b. Excess body weight

c. Climacteric complaints, circulatory or nervous

The implication of a proliferative smear in a postmenopausal women with oestrogen production was probably that it protects the patients against some facets of the oestrogen deficiency syndrome; on the other hand, this was a risk factor predisposing the women to a higher incidence of uterine bleeding and perhaps some neoplastic changes in certain target cell tissues.

Efstratiades et al (1982) carried out a cytohormonal evaluation of vaginal smears in three groups of women, all over the age of 50 years with menopause since at least one year. The observation of the three groups that is,

597 healthy women (controls), 134 cases of squamous cell carcinoma of cervix uteri and 167 patients of endometrial adenocarcinoma, revealed 4%, 6% and 12% smears respectively with unequivocal oestrogenic effect. It was concluded that increased oestrogenic activity in women more than one year after menopause, requires a thorough clinical investigation to exclude asymptomatic carcinoma of the cervix or the endometrium.

Phillis et al (1986) tried to compare the cytohormonal status of postmenopausal women with cancer to age matched controls. They found that epidermoid carcinoma was identified in 64 patients, with an average age 67 yrs and adenocarcinoma in 34 patients with an average age 69 yrs.

Among the evaluable cases with epidermoid carcinoma of the cervix, a high maturation was noted in 46% as compared to 11% in the matched controls. In addition, high maturation was observed in 69% of those patients with endometrial carcinoma as compared to 19% in the matched controls. None of the index cases were atrophic but 31% of control cases showed atrophy.

In cases with exogenous administration of oestrogen, three cases of endometrial carcinoma showed high maturation while in five control cases, none had a high maturation value.

These findings indicate that the difference in the cytohormonal status of patients with cervical carcinoma as compared to those without carcinoma, consequently alerts the cytologist to the fact that they should have been attentive to the smears showing high maturation in the postmenopausal women. This is because the patient in the group with high oestrogenic smears may harbour preneoplastic lesions or an occult genital tract cancer.

This point has also been noted by Rubio et al (1967), while studying the cytohormonal values (KPI) in cases of recurrent carcinoma.

They also noted that the cases of recurrent carcinoma showed high maturation value in 6.8% cases, which was confirmed by Liu and others workers.

Valenzuela et al (1993) conducted the "Progestin Challenge Test" in 157 postmenopausal women and compared the characteristics of the patients who bled with those who did not bleed. Results showed that in cases that bled, 14.01% were significantly and independently more overweight. They had higher levels of plasma estradiol and a clear presence of superficial cells in the vaginal smears and had been menopausal for fewer years than those who did not bleed. The test thus identifies women at risk from hormone related endometrial carcinoma.

Jakkola et al (2012) published the report on the results of their work, where they evaluated the association of postmenopausal Estradiol Protection Therapy (EPT) with the risk of precancerous tumours, squamous cell carcinoma and adenocarcinoma of the uterine cervix in women over the age of 50 years. These patients were undertreatment fromsix months to five years.

She found no evidence of association with precancerous lesions but the risk was decreased for squamous cell carcinoma and increased for adenocarcinoma when the use was prolonged over five years.

The idea of these studies was that hormones should be used with great care in postmenopausal women.Oestrogenic activity declines progressively with the passing years, and patients may progressively suffer from arthritis, hypertension, hypercholestremia, osteoporosis, and psychic disorders. In such cases oestrogen therapy is given to help the gradually failing oestrogen function. Most of the workers in this field have recommended that hormonal status should be checked before starting oestrogen therapy since moderate or high oestrogenic activity in an older patient is alarming and a signal of proliferative activity,which may lead to malignancy. Therefore cytohormonal evaluation is of great help before and after the oestrogen test and treatment.

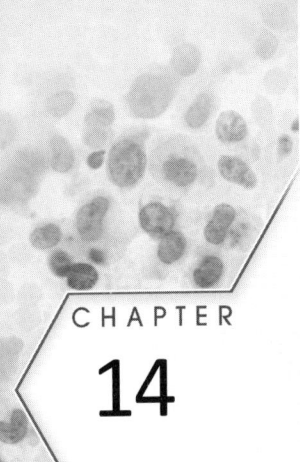

Techniques for Vaginal Smear Preparation and Staining

Exfoliative cytology is the study of cells which are shed off in the body cavities. For cytohormonal studies of the exfoliated vaginal cells, the following techniques are used.

1. Colpocytogram (vaginal smear study): For assessment of the cytohormonal values in cases where colpocytogram is contraindicated or cannot be done, the following two alternative techniques are available

2. Nymphocytogram (vulvar smear from the inner surface of labia minora)

3. Urocytogram–Urinary sediment–smear (morning specimen, preferably obtained through catheter)

Colpocytogram gives the best results as the vagina is the most sensitive indicator of the hormonal status in females. This is because the vagina, vulva and trigone of the bladder, all originate embryologically from the same source, that is, the urogenital sinus, thus providing identical results, with neglible differences. Hence in those circumstances, where a vaginal study on account of bleeding or infection cannot be carried out, a nymphocytogram or preferably a urocytogram can be used as a replacement.

1. **Colpocytogram:** Papanicolaou first studied the colpocytogram in 1925 in a pregnant woman, by collecting the posterior vaginal pool secretions with the help of a special pipette, which he designed himself and which was named after him as Papanicolaou's pipette.

The Papanicolaou pipette was a glass tube (later replaced by a plastic tube) with rounded edges on both sides, 15 cms in length having a bore of 0.5 cm. It was bent on one side a few centimetres before the end. The other end had a detachable rubber bulb (Fig. 14.1).

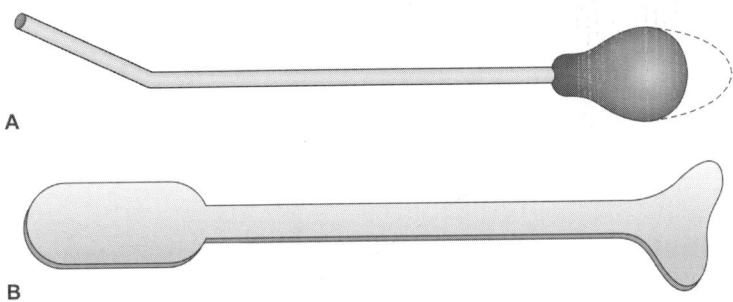

A

B

Fig. 14.1: Pap. Tube and Ayer's Spatula

Papanicolaou discovered the stain in 1942 and it was later modified by Traut in 1943. Papanicolaou first described the method of obtaining the posterior vaginal pool secretions and prepared it in the form of a blood smear, then stained it with the Papanicolaou stain.

Technique for the collection of the vaginal pool secretions: (Erica Wachtel 1969)

The fluid from the post vaginal pool is obtained by pushing lightly the Papanicolaou pipette with its attached rubber bulb into the vagina, when the patient is lying in the lithotomy position, and then allowing the pipette to glide into the post vaginal fornix (without the help of a speculum). The bulb is kept compressed until the tip of the pipette reaches the posterior fornix, then the compression is gradually released so that the contents of the aspirate are drawn into the pipette. The pipette is then drawn out and its material is pushed onto a grease free glass side and the smear is prepared like a thin blood smear.

The vaginal pool smear contains cells from the entire female genital tract, but being a stagnant fluid, with sometimes evidence of mild infection in a multigravida, it showed marked degenerative changes. Hence it was found unsuitable for cytohormonal evaluation after preliminary study by various workers.

Pundal (1959) expressed his opinion that blind collection of secretions from the posterior vaginal pool by means of a pipette had no value for the cytodiagnosis of pregnancy smears.

Paul K. Birtch (1961) also stated that "the vaginal pool smear offers a more confusing picture and is unreliable especially in pregnancy; because there is greater dilution, the cells are older, cytolysis is common and associated debris and concomitant vaginal and cervical infections are present to some degree in all cases." Therefore he preferred anterior vaginal wall smear and Pundal and Wachtel preferred smears from the upper one-third of the lateral vaginal wall for study. The anterior vaginal wall is less contaminated with infection, and lateral vaginal wall which is most sensitive to hormonal activity is preferred by all.

The smears could also be obtained with the help of Ayer's spatula or dry gloved finger or nonabsorbable cotton swabs. In these procedures, collection is to be done with the help of a dry vaginal speculum to avoid contamination from the cervix. We preferred collection by a dry gloved finger, asprepared by Dr Rizvi .*

*Dr R.Rizvi, (Gyaenocologist,J.N.M.C.) discovered a new method of preparation .

Technique: A drop of the material or deposit is put in the centre of a grease free glass slide with the help of dry gloved finger and is carried around it in circles till the material is exhausted.This was a better method of spreading the material for cytohormonal evaluation.

Inspite of the limitations of cytohormonal evaluation by the colpocytogram as a diagnostic tool of pregnancy, it still holds a greater promise for prognosis in the follow up of a normal pregnancy, threatened abortion and in the screening of the patients with disturbed pregnancy. In general, the advantage of estimating the hormonal activity by colposcopy is enhanced by the fact that vaginal epithelial cells respond earlier and with more sensitivity than the other methods of testing, that is, biological assays or chemical analysis.

For cytohormonal vaginal smear study, one should always ask the clinician for the patient's clinical data along with the following:

1. Precautions to be taken before the smear test

2. Last menstrual period and the normal menstrual pattern

3. Exact site from which the smear is obtained

4. Therapy details and last dose of hormone taken by patient on date

5. If the patient is under hormone therapy, details of drugs and their doses.

The vaginal smear, collected from different sites show variable results, based on the sensitivity of the site for the hormone action (LIU-1961). Further the smears should be repeated from the same site (i.e. first smear site) and if possible should be obtained by the same person. Staining of smears is done by the Papanicolaou method.

2. **Nymphocytogram:** This is the study of hormonal changes reflected in the smear, obtained from the inner surface of the labia minora.

The reports of nymphocytogram are few. DelCastillo and Vadela (1966) were the first ones to study it, and later reports were of Dennerstein (1968), Vadela and DelCastillo (1969), Tozzini et al (1971), Bazovsky (1973). Pinto et al (1968) were the first ones to discuss a comparative study of all the three techniques, that is, colpocytogram, nymphocyogram and urocytogram use in pregnancy applying EI and KPI indices. Shamim, Khan and Rizvi (1977) carried out a detailed study of hormonal cytology in pregnancy with a comparative statistical evaluation of colpo, nympho, and uro–cytograms, based on the indices - KPI, MV, CCI and FCI along with bacterial flora and cytolysis details.

Pinto et al were of the opinion that vulvar cytology is a good alternative to vaginal cytology while Shamim et al found that urocytogram appears to be the best alternative especially in a serial study where the patient is bleeding or suffering from infection. Although the urinary sediment smear preparation is tedious and time consuming, the catheter specimen is easy to collect and is completely free of blood and infection in disorders of pregnancy such as a threatened abortion. As the nymphocytogram normally shows a high KPI in the first trimester of pregnancy, it may not be possible to use it as a prognostic tool for cytohormonal assessment in threatened abortion.

Technique for Nymphocytogram

The lips of labia minora are separated and with the dry, gloved, right index finger, containing a drop of fixative on it, a smear is obtained from the inner surface of labia minora and is prepared on a grease free glass slide.

Staining of the smear is done by the Papanicolaou method.

3. **Urocytogram:** This is the study of urinary sediment smears, prepared either from freshly voided morning specimen or preferably from a catheterised specimen in case of vaginal bleeding and infection in disturbed pregnancy. This method was first described by Papanicolaou in 1948 in a catheterised specimen for the diagnosis of pregnancy, following a study by Biot and Belteron (1944). Later delCastillo, Argonz and Galli Mainini (1948, 1949) reported its parallelism with the vaginal smear. Lencioni published some preliminary reports and finally proved that the urocytogram is very useful in evaluating ovarian function and hormonal treatment. In 1965 Lencioni reported that in normal pregnancy there is a relationship of urinary and vaginal cytology with the urinary oestriol and pregnandid estimations.

Lencioni (1969) described a special technique for staining the urinary sediment which is quick and simple, and the training for interpretation of smears by this technique requires a relatively short period of time. In normal pregnancies, the information obtained is comparable to that from the vaginal smear.

The technique for the preparation of urinary sediment smears as outlined by Lencioni 1969 is as follows: A freshly voided morning specimen or catheterised specimen of urine is collected in a clean test tube. The smear is prepared by the following method.

1. 20 C.C. of urine is taken in a conical glass tube and centrifuged at 800 rpm for 5 minutes

2. The supernatant is decanted and 20CC of Ringer solution *(diluted in water 50: 50) added to it. Shake the tube to dissolve the sediment at the bottom

3. This is centrifuged again for 5 minutes at 800 rpm and then the supernatant is decanted

4. Extract the sediment that is sticking to the bottom of the tube by means of a Pasteur pipette

5. Push the sediment material onto the slide and prepare a smear

6. Allow the smear to air dry. (No fixation is required)

Lencioni (1969) used the following special technique for the staining of these air dried smears

Haemotoxylin – Shorr's staining for urinary sediment smear

a. Hydrate the material by dipping the slide in distilled water – 2 minutes

b. Place in the Harris Haemotoxylin stain – 2 minutes

c. Rinse in distilled water – 2 dips

d. Place into the ammonium Hydroxide alcholic solution – ½ minute

e. Wash gently with water

f. Place in 2% acetic acid in 30% alcohol – 2 minutes

g. Place in 2% acetic acid in 70% alcohol – 2 minutes

h. Place in Shorr's stain-4 minutes

i. Wash gently with water

j. Then dehydrate by rinsing with 2% acetic acid in 70% alcohol

k. Dehydrate in 95% alcohol with 2% acetic acid

l. Finally rinse in absolute alcohol. Now clear with xylene and Mount in Canada Balsam

Note: This is a good technique for pregnancy smears (which have quite a heavy exfoliate).*Ringer solution disolves the mucous and cellular debris, commonly found in late pregnancy.

In cases of poor cellularity like ameno-rrhoea or in girls at puberty, it is convenient to shorten this process by omitting (b, c, d and e) steps.

The other good technique described in the literature is by O Morchoe and O Morchoe (1967) and Nyklicek (1968). Both the workers used centrifugation at a higher speed for a longer period, without washing in Ringer's solution.

We have used Lencioni's method (1969) and found it most suitable for research as well as in routine practice.

Shorr's Stain for Vaginal and Vulval Smears (1941):

This is a simple technique, most suitable for hormonal assessment. It is quick and time saving. Shorr's stain is supposed to be a better stain for studying Eosinophilic (EI) Index in hormonal cytology (European workers preferred it). Smears are fixed in 95% alcohol.

Shorr's Technique for Staining Smears

1. Smears are passed through graded concentrations of alcohol for hydration.

2. Stain in Harris – Haematoxylin for 15 minutes.

3. Smears are passed through 70% alcohol with ammonia 13% by volume.

4. Stain in Shorr's stain for 10 minutes.

5. Dehydrate and clean and mount in Canada Balsam.

Shorr's Stain Preparation

1. Biebrich Scarlet – 1.5 gm

2. Orange – G – 0.5 gm

3. Analine Blue – 1.25 gm

4. Fastgreen – 0.375 gm

5. Phosphotungstic Acid – 1.25 gm
6. Phosphomolybdic Acid – 1.25 gm
7. Absolute Alcohol – 250 ml
8. Glacial Acetic Acid – 5 ml

Note: This stain gives a spectrum of colour to the cytoplasm according to the cell types: blue, green, pink.

Technique for staining of the cytoplasmic lipid granules in the vaginal epithelial cells. (Maillet et al 1978)

a. Baker's Method (1957)

Baker's Solution for fixation of smear
1. 90 CC of Double distilled water
2. 10 CC of 40% formaldehyde
3. 3.1 gm of anhydrous calcium chloride

The smears soon after the preparation are fixed for an average time, that is, 48 hrs in the Barker's solution.

b. Staining (By Lilles Method) for Granules

Stain Using oil Red O. (Gurr Ltd) in Isopropyl acid and counter stain with Light Green.

Result: Granules of Deep Purple colour in the cytoplasm of vaginal epithelial cells, show specific pattern in pre and post ovulatory phases as these are sensitive to hormones. Details of the pattern are given in the chapter on Menstrual cycle (Table 7.2).

Papnicolaou Method of Staining

By Papanicolaou and Traut 1943.The method of staining is similar for vaginal, vulval, and oral smear.

Anderson et al (1969) have reported the effect of oestrogen therapy in postmenopausal women on the oral mucosa and compared it with their vaginal cytology for general hormonal evaluation. It can be utilized for serial smears, if functioning vaginal epithelium is not available.

In 1972 Hugoson et al studied the value of cytohormonal assessment of pregnancy in oral and vaginal smears. The vaginal epithelium showed a characteristic pattern of the normal pregnancy smear which indicated that hormonal balance was normal, while at the same time oral mucosa showed a constant cell picture without any significant variation in the distribution of the different type of cells.Therefore the oral mucosa smears cannot be used for hormonal assessment in pregnancy.

Papanicolaou Staining

It is a polychromatic stain, which gives a spectrum of colours (green – blue – pink and orange) to the cytoplasm depending on the maturity of cells. It indicates the effect of hormone by the different colours. In addition it gives a clear nuclear staining which in addition to the hormonal effect on cytoplasm, reveals the profile of the DNA (Nucleus).

The stains required are:

a. Harris – Haemotoxylin
b. Orange – G
c. Polychrome stain EA – 36 or EA 65 or EA – 50.

Preparation of the Stain

Haematoxylin (Powder) – 1 gm
95% alcohol (ethyl) – 10 ml
Potassium alum – 20 gm
Distilled water – 200 ml
Mercuric oxide – 0.5 gm

Potassium alum is dissolved in water with the aid of heat; when the alum is fully in solution, Haematoxylin which is already dissolved in alcohol, is added to it. The mixture is rapidly brought to boiling point and mercuric oxide is added cautiously. When the solution turns a dark purple colour, it s removed from the heat and rapidly cooled. It has been found in practice that on addition of 4% glacial acetic acid, the staining of the nuclei is improved.

Orange G

Orange G – 100 ml (0.5% solution ethyl alcohol) Phosphotangstic Acid – 0.015 gm.

Polychrome Stain-EA-36

Light Green (SF yellow)
0.1% solution in 95% Enylalcohol – 45 ml.
Bismark Brown
0.5% (solution) in 95% Ethyl alcohol – 10 ml

Eosin Yellow

0.5% solution in 95% alcohol – 45 ml
Phosphotungstic Acid – 0.2 gm
(as mordant)
Lithium Carbonate (Saturated aqueous solution)– 1 drop

Note: All these stains can be easily dissolved in water as 10% solution aqueous solution. Keep these in stock, while using these as a stain, dilute with alcohol.

Staining Technique

1. Remove the slides from the fixative and pass through the descending alcohol strengths (80%, 70%,50%, 30%) and then through water for hydration
2. Stain in Harris Haematoxylin for 3 minutes (approximately)
3. Rinse in tap water
4. Differentiate it in 0.5% aqueous Hydrochloric Acid until the cytoplasm of cells is decolourised and the nuclei retain the stain (Check through microscope)
5. Rinse in tap water and 'blue'it in ammoniated water until the desired (bluing) staining density is reached
6. Wash in running tap water for 5 minutes
7. Pass through ascending grades of alcohol strengths(50%, 70%, 80% and 2 changes of 95% alcohol)
8. Stain in orange G approx 2 minutes
9. Rinse in 2 changes of 95% alcohol
10. Stain in EA – 36 for approximately 2 – 4 minutes until the desired intensity of colour has been reached
11. Rinse in 2 changes of 95% alcohol
12. Drain, clear in Xylol and mount in neutral mountant (DPX)

Note: I have given the details of the technique, which we were using in our laboratory of JNMC, Department of Pathology.

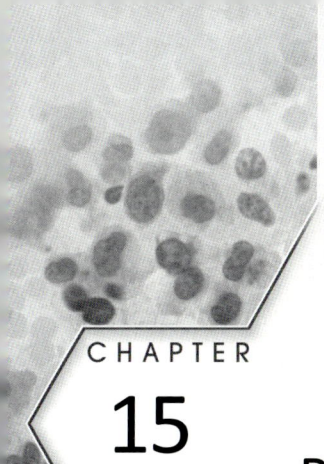

Introduction to the Chapter on Phase Contrast Direct Microscopy

Role of Phase Contrast Direct Microscopy in Daily Gynecologic Practice
By
Giovanni Miniello
Professor, Dept Obstet Gynecol, University of Bari, Italy
- International Consultant of Colposcopy for the United Nations
- Trainer of The International Agency for Research on Cancer
- Visiting Professor of Colposcopy and Uro-Gynaecologic Cytologyin different foreign Universities

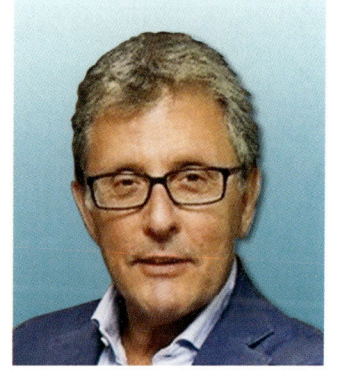

Phase-contrast microscopy was developed in 1935 by a Dutch physicist Fritz Zernike, Nobel laureate in 1953, based on Ernst Abbe's studies. (Fig. 15.1a and b)

At the beginning of 1940's Michel observed by Ph equipment and documented for the first time the complete procedure of cell division.

In 1943, Zinser extended the cytodiagnostic possibilities by the use of phase-contrast microscopy which enabled the study of live, unstained cells; but only in 1949 this technique was introduced into Gynecology by Runge, Voge, Haselmann and Zinser himself.

In 1969 Peter Stoll and Gisela Dallenbach-Hellweg produced the first work of phase-contrast microscopy by Springer-Verlag Publisher, followed by the Atlas of Miniello in 1994 by CIC Edizioni Internazionali.

Phase contrast microscopy is slowly gaining popularity among Gynaecologists. However, up till today it has not still assumed the role in practice that its diagnostic potential and its value in screening deserves.

In many centres it is the practice to use wet mount or direct microscopy as an extension of the routine gynecologic checkup, in order to obtain more complete information about the vaginal flora.

Vaginal discharge and cervical secretion are collected by swabs, spatulas or other appropriate devices (Fig. 15.2).

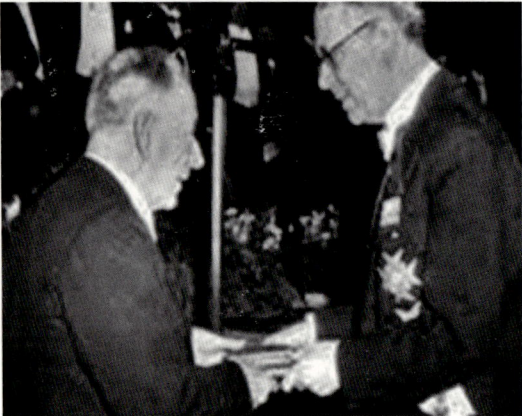

Fig. 15.1a

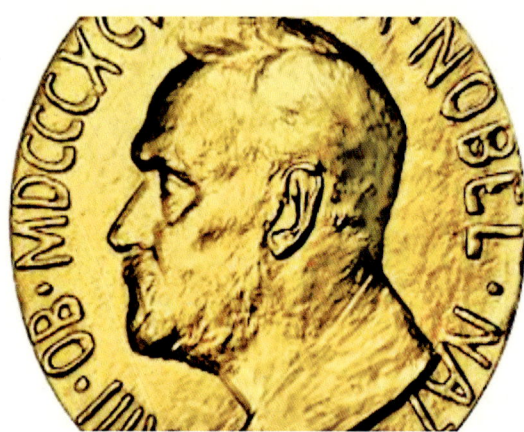

Fig. 15.1b

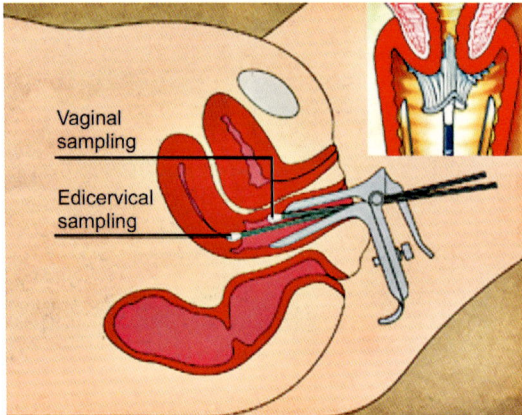

Vaginal sampling

Edicervical sampling

Fig. 15.2:

The device is immediately and gently rubbed in a drop of saline, previously applied on a microscope slide.

Soon after the specimen is mounted with a coverslip and the sample is thus ready to be examined by a Ph microscope, without fixation or staining.

The tonality of the pictures is due to a stained glass placed on the filter holder because, due to the physical peculiarity of Ph microscopy, monochromatic light enables optimum contrast.

A wet mount can provide immediate information about:

1. Hormonal condition
2. Cervico-vaginal microbiology
3. Cell changes induced by pathogens
4. Cell-mediated immunity
5. Stages of metaplastic process
6. Atypical cells

In this article I will discuss only Hormonal condition.

Direct microscopy has been confirmed to be a precious diagnostic tool in the evaluation of the hormonal milieu at different ages of a woman.

The hormonal stimulation on the vaginal epithelium is responsible for the prevalence of different types of cells in the vaginal smear. (Fig. 15.3)

This peculiar cell distribution characterizes four cytologic patterns.

In childhood, usually the smear is atrophic. At times the girl child may complain of a mucoid discharge and a state of constant wetness. If the smear is found to be oestrogenic, it may indicate the possibility of precocius puberty or an oestrogen producing ovarian tumour. (Fig. 15.4a and b)

Cytologic evidence may appear long before Radiological evidence or MR findings.

The onset of puberty can be confirmed when there is thelarche and adrenarche.

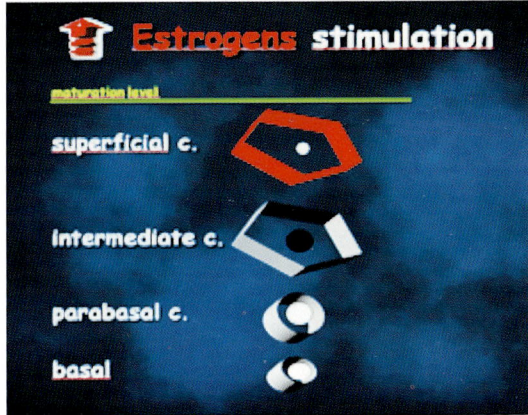

Fig. 15.3

During child bearing years, a woman's smears will depend upon ovulation. Cytolytic smear is noted when the intermediate cells are fragmented and the smear appears "dirty". It may indicate the presence of Progesterone and or androgens. It is seen in late secretory phase, during pregnancy or when the woman is on oral contraceptives (Fig. 15.5a).

Cytolitic smear observed in the advanced proliferative phase may indicate an excess of androgens.

If in the late secretory phase, an oestrogenic smear is seen it may indicate absence of ovulation or defective luteal phase. (Fig. 15.5b) Smears taken in 1st half (Fig. 15.6a and b) and repeated in 2nd half (Fig. 15.7a and b) of cycle may give a clue to diagnosis.

Smear showing good cytolytic patterns indicates good progestrone activity (Fig. 15.8a and b) and defective luteal phase will show poor cytolosis and presence of oestrogen active cells.

In cases of amenorrhoea, an atropic smear will indicate poor activity of hypothalamus and pituitary or ovarian failure (Fig. 15.9).

However, if there are cyclic changes in the vaginal epithelium, it can be presumed that ovarian function is normal but it is the endometrium which is not responding.

Hormonal Cytology is particularly important in perimenopausal women.

The presence of normal endometrial cells, except around peri-menstrual period, is abnormal. It is seen in intrauterine device users. (Fig. 15.10) If the woman is past 40 years of age, it may warrant additional investigation to exclude endometrial hyperplasia (Fig. 15.11).

Post menopause, the ovarian function ceases. When the smear becomes atrophic and inflammatory, the woman will complain of irritation, discharge and pain. She will benefit from hormone therapy.

During therapy wih oestrogens after menopause (HRT) vaginal hormonal cytology is useful to assess response. When highly

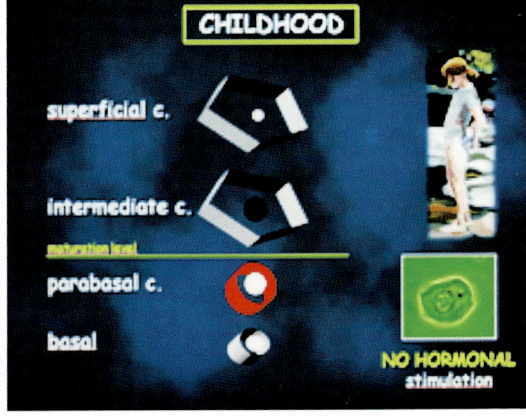

Fig. 15.4a

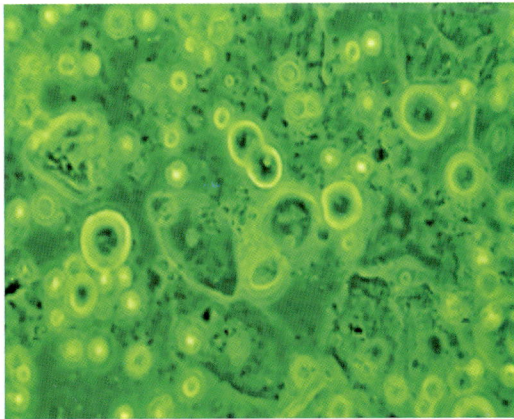

Fig. 15.4b: Atrophic smear

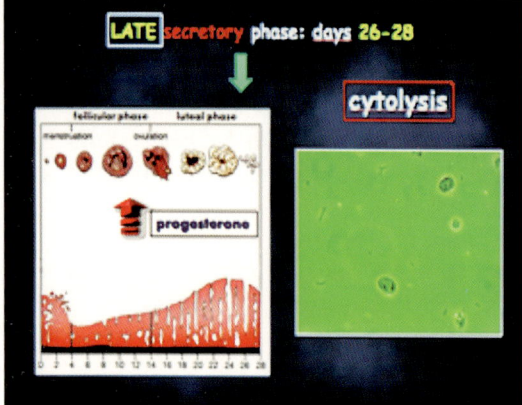

Fig. 15.5a

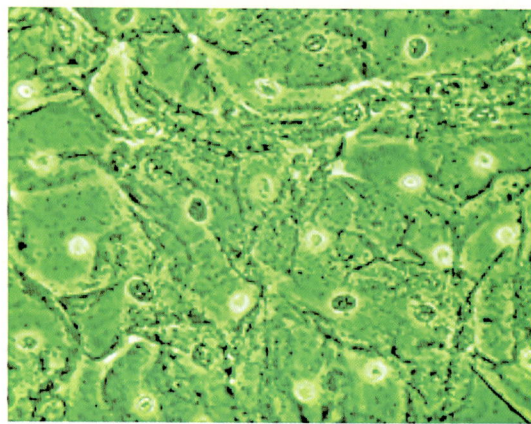

Fig. 15.5b

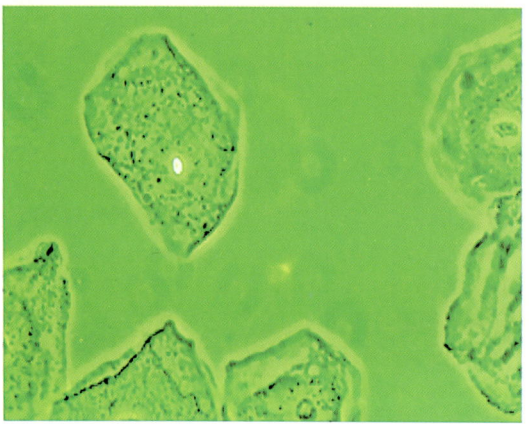

Fig. 15.6a: Estrogenic smear

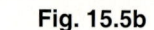

Fig. 15.6b: Estrogenic Smear

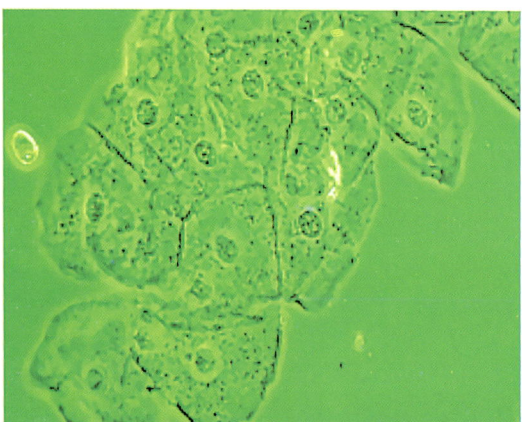

Fig. 15.7a: Progestinic Smear

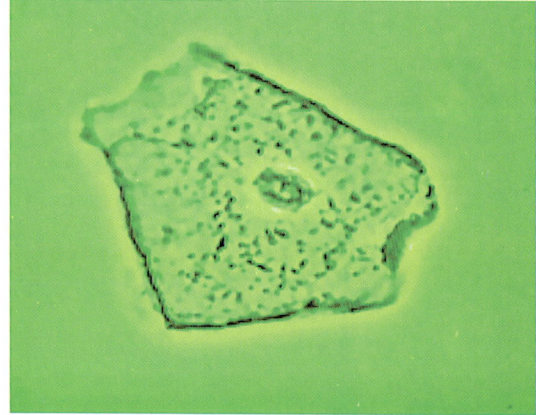

Fig. 7b: Progesterone Effect

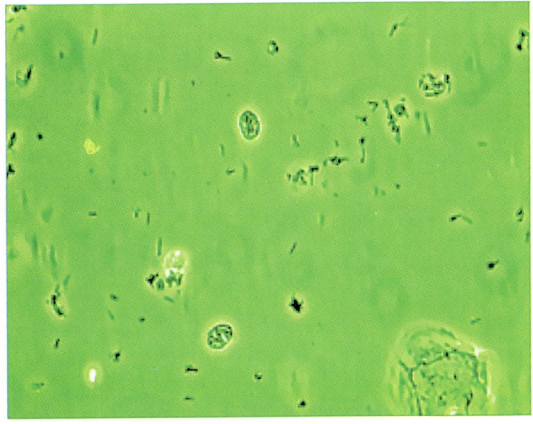

Fig 15.8a: Cytolytic Smear

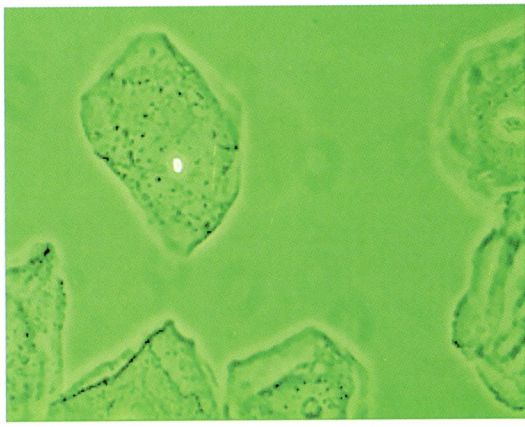

Fig. 15.8b: Endometrial dysfunction

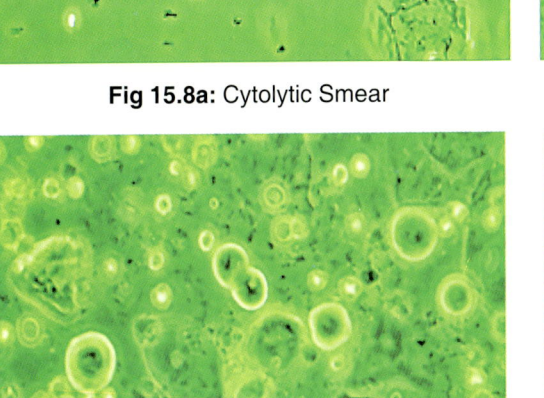

Fig. 15.9: Hypothalamic and pituitary defector ovarian failure

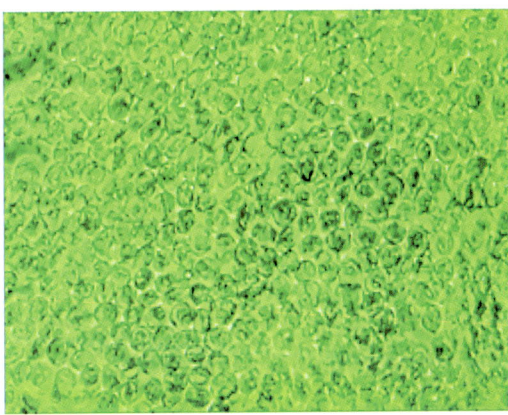

Fig. 15.10: Perimenstrual period Ovulation–IUD

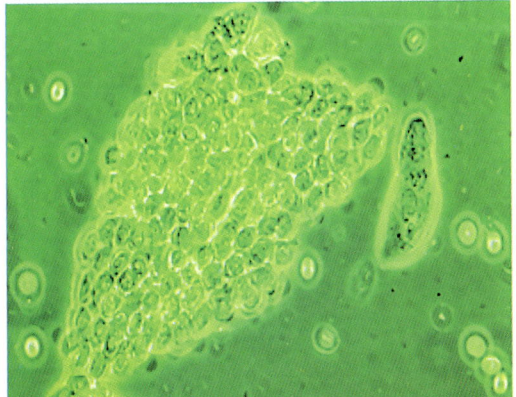

Fig. 15.11: Additional diagnostic evaluationis mandatory (glandular hyperplasia)

oestrogenic smear is noted, the amount of oestrogen given orally needs to be reduced. In case of persistent higly oestrogenic smear additional diagnostic work up is required to exclude tumors of breast, endometrium or ovaries (Fig. 15.12).

Conclusion

In clinical practice, hormonal cytology can give a good idea of which hormones are acting on the cervico-vaginal epithelium. This in turn will indicate which investigations should be undertaken before initiating therapy. Furthur hormone therapy can best be monitored by its effect on the epithelium. Phase Contract

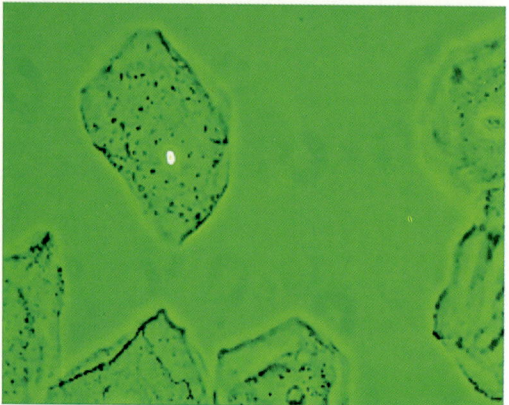

Fig. 15.12: Additional diagnostic evaluation is mandatory(tumors of breast, endometrium and ovaries, long-term treatment with tranquillizers)

Microscopy if introduced in clinical practice will help the Gynaecologist in treating women of all ages with evidence based data to correct the endocrinological pathologics.

REFERENCES

1. MINIELLO G : Citogramma Vaginale-Vaginal Cytogram. CIC Edizioni Internazionali, 1994.
2. MINIELLO G. Colposcopia e Microscopia a fresco–Colposcopy and Phase Contrast Microscopy. CIC Edizioni Internazionali, 1998.
3. MINIELLO G. Le Micosi Vaginali in microscopia a fresco. Vaginal Fungal Infec-tions by phase contrast microscopy. CIC Edizioni Internazionali, 2001–2012.
4. MINIELLO G., SARAIYA U. Color Atlas of Cytology and Colposcopy. CBS Publishers, New Delhi, 1999.
5. SARAIYA UB, MINIELLO G. Atlas of Cytology and Colposcopy. Jaypee Brothers Medical Publishers, 2009.
6. SARAIYA UB, MINIELLO G. Citologìa y Colposcopìa en la Pràctica Ginecològica. Jaypee Brothers Medical Publishers, 2010.
7. STOLL P, DALLENBACH-HELLWEG G: Cytology in Gynecological Practice. An Atlas of Phase Contrast Microscopy-Gynäkologische Vitalzytologie in der Praxis. Atlas der Phasenkontrastmikroskopie. Springer-Verlag, 1993.

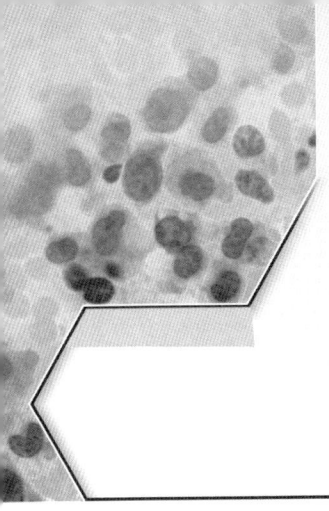

Bibliography

1. Abrams, RY., and Abrams, J., Actacytol Philad. 6:359–364 :1962.

2. Aktinson, W.B. and Engle E.T.: Endocrinology, 40:327–333: 1947.

3. Allen E: Am. J. Anat., 30:297–371; 1922.

4. Anupama, H., Sailaga, G., Sudhakar, R., Reddy, C. J. Obstet and Gynaecol, India, pp 83–85:2011

5. Anderson,W.R., Belding, J., and Pixley, E.: Acta. Cytol.13:81–83,1969.

6. Ault, K.A. Infectious Diseases Obstetric. Gynaecol. 2006.

7. Ayre W.B., J.Clin.Endocr.11:103–109,1951.

8. B.R. Series – Biology and Histopathology 4th Edition. 2002. pp 258–264.

9. Baker: Nature, 80:947; 1957.

10. Bamford, S.B., Mitchell, G.W Jr. Bardawil, W.A., Claire Cassin. Acta Cytol, 11:257–261; 1967

11. Barbour, E.M.: J. Obst, Gynec Brit Comm, 68 662–667;1961.

12. Batrinos M.L., Eustratiades MG., and Kalliga, B. Fertility and Sterility 20:590–598; 196913).

13. Batrinos, M.L. andEustratiades M.G., Acta Cytol;16:376–380;1972.

14. Batrinos, M.L.: IATRIKI– 13: 161–180, 1968.

15. Bazovsky, P., et al: Cesk Gynekol;38: 134–135, 1973 (LZR).

16. Bardawill, W.A; Mitchell, G.W; Jr. McKeogh, R.P. and Merchant, D.J: Am. J. Obst. and Gynec; 84: 1283–1299, 1962.

17a. Bercovici, B., D1iamant, Y, and Polishuk, W.Z., Acta Cytol, 17:67–72; 1973.

17b. Bernstien, J.B., and Rak off, A.E.; Vaginal infections, infestations and discharges. Blackiston company, New York pp 99,1955.

18. Bhose, Chowdhury L.N., , J.R and Bose, S.,J. Ind. Med. Ass., 57: 328–330, 1971

19. Bibbo et al Acta Cytol 13: 260–1969.

20. Biot, R., Y Beltran, Nunez, R., 1944 Sem Med Buenos Aires 2:532–535.

21. Birtch, P.K.: Cl. Obst. Gynec 4: 1062–1074; 1961.

22. Bonime, R.G., Am, J. Obst. Gynec., 60: 1306-1314.

23. Boschann H.W.: Acta Cytol 12:112; 1968.

24. Boschann, H.W. (1960) Quoted by Erica Wachtel,"Exfoliative Cytology in gynaecological Practice" 1969.

25. Bose, S, Chowdhury, J.R., Bhose, L.N. and Guhathakurata, S; Reports of Sixth World Congress of Gynaec and Obst, Chicago, 1970, Baltimore. The William and Wilkins Co.

26. Bourg, R., Pundal J.P. Acta gym obst Histopath. IUS 1951, page 621.

27. Bourg, R., VanMeensel and Lambert Annals d' Endorinologic, 2:262; 1953.

28. Bret, J.A., Legros, R., Coupez F.J; Acta Cytol 3: 323–329; 1959.

29. Britsch, Ch, J. and H.A. Azar, Am J ObstGynec 85: 989–993; 1963.

30. Brown, W.E. and Bradbury, J.T.: J. Clin. Endorcinol. 9:725; 1949.

31. Brown, J.B; Mac Leod, S.C;Macnaughtan, C; Smith, M.A. and Smyth, B.; J. Endocrinol. 42:5;1968.

32. Brown, J.B; Lancet, 270: 704;1956.

33. Brunori, I.L. (1965) Quoted Stone etal 1967.

34. Butler, E.B. and Taylor D.S: Actacytol; 17: 237–240; 1973.

35. Cathernine M., Keebler, C.T. and Wied G.L. Acta Cytol 18: 482–493, 1974.

36. Cieciura,L., and Wisniowska,A; Ginek Polish, 41:191–197; 1970.

37. Charles, D.L; etal: Am. J.Obst Gynec.; 94:527–533; 1966.

38. De Allende, I.L.C., and Orias, O.,(1950) "Cytology of Human Vagina, Newyork Hoebar pp 184–225.

39. De Laguna, J.G., Guarcia, G., Urrutia,A., M., Graham, J.C., and Mungvia, H. (1958). QuotedbyWachtel, E; (1969 pp 63.

40. Dehnhard, F; etal (1973,1975) Quotedby Ortneretal 1977 pp 429

41. DeBrux, J.A. and Del Sace: Masson, Paris (1958, in French language), Quoted by Sonek (1967) p.p 44.

42. Dudkiewicz, J.: Ginek. Pol 39: 989 – 993; 1968.

43. Delcastillo, E.B., Argonz, J., and Galli, Mainini, C., J. Clin. Endocrine. 8: 76-87; 1948 and 9: 1362–1371; 1949.

44. DelCastillo, E.B., and Videla, Acta. Cytol., 10: 236–237; 1966.

45. Dellepiane, G.,Acta Cytol, 3: 282; 1959.

46. Demol and Movrozies; – Quoted by Ruiz M., 1968. pp. 113.

47. DeNeef, J.C., Clinical Endrorine Cytology. Hoeber Med. Div. New York, Harper of Row. 1965.

48. Dennerstein, G.J. Obstel Gynaec. Brit Cwth 75: 603-609; 1968.

49. Dexeus, Jr., Fernandez-cid, A., and Carrera, J.M. Acta Ginec (Madrid) 17: 369-378; 1966.

50. Dudkiewicz, J.: Acta Cytol 21: 578-587; 1977.

51. Dudkiewicz, J.: Slaska Akad Med. Katowice 1974 (Thesis)

52. Dudkiewicz, J., Ginek. Polish., 39:989–993;1968.

53. Efstratiades, M., Tamva kopoulou, E. Papatheodorou, B., Batrinos, M., Acta Cytol 26: 126–128; 1982.

54. Ebner,V.H.(1954) Quoted by Maillet 1978

55. Engel, L.L., Human Ovulation Boston, Little Brown and Co. 1965)

56. Farber, E., Sternberg, W.H. and Dunlap, C.E. Endrokr. Pol. 16: 55–62, 1965.

57. Ferriman, D and Purdie, A.W.: (1965) Brit med. J. (ii) 1969.

58. Ferin, J., Acta.Cytol;12:117;1968

59. Ferin J. (Louvian, Belguim) Acta Cytol 3:234–35; 1959.

60. Fletcher, P.F: Am J. Obst. And Gynec, 39:562; 1940.

61. Ford, C.E., and Jones, K.W.: Lancet 1: 711; 1959.

62. Frost, J.K., "Gynaecologic and Obstetric Pathology" Chapter 35, P–595, 1958, Ed by Novak, London, W.B. Sounders.

63. Gaudefroy, M., and VanMeensel: Quoted by Robert E.L. et al Obst and Gynac 17:1961.

64. Gaudefroy, M.ActaCytol; 3:228; 1959.

65. Gaudefroy, M. (1955) Quoted by Ferin, J., 1968, pp117.

66. Gomez LM; Ma, Y. Ho Cetal; Human Reproduction: 23:709;2008

67. Gaudefroy, M.," J. Sc. Med. Lille 68: 202; 1950.

68. Garud, AM., Saraiya, U.B., etal. J.Obstet and Gynec. India Vol.xxviii:No3:436-442;1978.

69. Gorden, H.W; A.M.Rywlin; H. Sussman and PMarwan: Am. J.Obst. and Gynec., 94:524–526; 1966.

70. Gompel,CandPundal ,J.P.;Acta.Cytol. 1:83; 1957 (Philadelphia).

71. Hammand, D.O.: Acta Cytol 9: 340-343; 1965.

72. Hindman, W.M., Schwalenberg, R.R. and Efstation,T.Acta Cytol 6: 365–369, 1962.

73. Hermont, P.L., Kechelava, S., Lowery, C.L., et al Human Pathology 29:170; 1998.

74. Hertig, A.T., Ward Burdick Lecture., Am J.Cl. Path. 47:249–268;1967

75. Hochsteadt, B., Lange, W., and Spira, H.: J. Obstet. Gynaec Brit. Colth 67: 102, 1960.

76. Hopman, B.C.: Acta Cytol 3: 291–297; 1959.

77. Hugoson, A., Winberg, E. and Angstrom, T., Acta Cytol;16:111–116;1972.

78. Iffy, L., Obstet. and Gynec; 26:490–498;1

79. International Academy of Cytology – 1958.

80. Jakkola et al: Int J. Cancer 19:257-271, 2012.

81. Jing, B.J., Kaufman, R.H. and Franklin, R.R. Am. J. Obst Gynaec.;99:546–550;1967

82. Joshi, J., Saraiya, U.B., and Fernandes, W., Proceeding of Ind.Ac. Cyt.pp.95–101;1971

83. Kamnitzer, MB: Acta Cytol, 3: 264; 1959 (Philadephia)

84. Klopper, A and Billewic, W., J. Obstet. Gynace, Brit Cwlth: 70: 1024, 1963.

85. Kaufman, R.H., Jing, B.J. and Franklin, R.R., Gynec. 34:396; 1969

86. Khan Ansar A.,Saeed Ahmad., and Rizvi Ruqqia.ActaCytol. 20:347–48;1976)

87. a. Langreder, W., Arch Gynak 183: 304, 1953.
    b. Langreder, W.and Merker, H. (1954), Quoted by Von Haam p326; 1961

88. Leeton, J. : Acta Cytol. 11:410-414; 1967.

89. Leeton, J.:J. Obst. and Gynaec. Brit. Cwith., 70:46;1963.

90. Lemberg – Siegfried, S., Stamm, O., and De Watteville, H., Presse. Med., 63:1558–1560, 1955.

91. Lencioni, L.J., Pocorone, R., Beligan L.T. and Beli, R.R.: Medicna (Buenos Aires) 15:71; 1955.

92. Lencioni, J., Luis, M. Martinez Amezaga and Victor, S. Lo Bianco: Acta Cytol 13: 279-287; 1969.

93. Lencioni, L.J; El. Urocytograma. Editorial Mediea, Panamericana 2nd Edition. Buenos Aires, 1963

94. Lencioni, L.J., Lo Bianco, V.S., Martinez Amezaga, l.a. and Badano, H; Amer. J. Obstet. Gynec. 91:1112–1122;1965 .

95. Lichtfuss, CP Acta Cytol 3:247–251; 1959

96. Lille's method of oil red staining.

97. Liu.W., Cancer.8:779-784;1955

98. Llusia, J.B., Van Keep P.A.: Actacytol 21:18-21.1977.

99. Luksch, F., Acta cytol 12: 98; 1968.

100. Loraine, J.A.: The clinical application of Hormone assay (1958) Liviving. Stone. Edinburgh.

101. MacRac, D.J., Acta Cytol (Balt) 11:45; 1967.

102. MacRae, D.J., Irani, J.B., Bowler,R.G. and Longhurst P.L., J. Obstel. Gynec. Brit. Comm 71:586–598; 1964.

103. Magie, T.P. Acta Cytol: 179-180; 1967.

104. Maillet, M., Dominique, J. Chiarasini., Etienne Cava, and Etienne Fournier; Acta Cytoli: 22; 479, 1978.

105. Malek J; Jitra, Kobilkoval, Enzen Cech; Dobramil Kuzel, Ata Cytol 11:444–448; 1967.

106. Masin, F. and Masin, M., Acta Cytol 8:263-269; 1964.

107. Masukawa, T., Obst and Gynec 16: 407–413; 1960.

108. Matter, R.: Gynaecologia, 139: 227–229; 1959.

109. McLennon, M. J., and McLennan, C.E.: Acta Cytol, 19: 431–433; 1975.

110. Meisels, A.,-Acta Cytol: 12:101; 1968.

111. Miesels, A.,-Acta Cytol; 113249; 1967.

112. Miesels, A. Acta Cytol. 10: 376–382; 1966.

113. Mills, I.H. and Wilson R.J.: Proc. Roy. Soc. Med 62:26; 1969.

114. Mills, I.H., Brooks, R.V., and Prunti, FTG 1962, Edited A.R. Currie et al Edinburgh and London, page 204.

115. Misra, S., Do Rosoario, Y.P. and Heera, P. J. Obstet gynec. India 10:443–447; 1969.

116. Mitra, R., Lahari, V.L. and Chowdhery, M; Acta. Cytol. 24:587;1974 and 25:194;1975.

117. Miniello, G. and Saraiya, U., Colour Atlas of Cytology and Colposcopy 1999,pp28. C.B.S. Publisher, Delhi.

118. Muth, H., Acta Cytol 4:151–152, 1960.

119. Navab, A., Koss, L.G. and La Due, J.S.: JAM Med Ass. 194: 30; 1965.

120. Neighburgs, H.E. and Greenbalt, R.B.; South Med. J.41:972;1948.

120. Neighburgs, H.E; Brit. J. Obst. Gynec., 54:653–656;1947.

122. Nelson, D., Holmquist and Danos Marion Acta Cytol,11:262–266;1967

123. Nesbitt,R.E.L.,Jr.Rogelio,G.,andRome,D.S; Obst. Gynee, 17: 2-8; 1961.

124. Neustaedter, T. and Mackenezie L.L.:1961 Am. J. Obstet and Gyne 47:81–92; 1944.

125. Noble, M.J.D. and M.E. Ahwood: J Obst Gynee, Brit Emp. 65: 64, 1958.

126. Nunez-clavera, J.A., Ruiz, M.L.: Acta Ginee (Madrid) 19: 639–654; 1968.

127. Nyklicek, O.,: Acta Cytol 12: 140; 1968.

128. Nyklicek, O.,: Acta Cytol; 16: 48–50; 1972.

129. Nyklicek, O.,: Gyanecologia (Basal) 131: 173 –178; 1951.

130. O'Morcheo, F.J. and Omorchoe, C.C.C.: Acta Cytol 11:145, 1967.

131. Ohlenroth, G. and Severin G.,: Geburtsh Frauenheilk, 27: 869-878; 1967.

132. Openion Poll on Cyt. Terminology: Acta Cytol, 2: 63–129; 1958.

133. Ortner, A., et al 1974, 1975 – Qoted by Ortner 1977.

134. 1Ortner, A., Klammar, J., Gier, W.,: Acta Cytol 21: 429-431, 1977.

135. Osmond – Clarke,F., and Murry M Brit. Med. J. Nov 9: 1172-1174; 1963.

136. Palliez, R., Dellecour, M., Monier, J.C. and Begveri, F., Gynec. and Obstet. 67:437–444;1968.

137. Pandit A.A.and Kalgutkar A.K.,Postgrad. Med. 32:210;1986.

138. Papazov. D.: Acta. Anat: 6:621; 1965.

139. Papanicolaou, G.NAm. J. of Anat 52:519–637; 1933.

140. Papanicolaou, G.N., Atlas on exfoliative Cytology. Cambridge, Mass. Harvard University Press 1657, G VII.

141. Papanicolaou, G.N. and Shorr, E.: Am J. Obst and Gynaec;31:806–831;1936.

142. Papanicolaou, G.N. and Trant H.F.: The common wealth fund New York (1943).

143. Papanicolaou, G.N.,: Proc. Soc. Exper. Biol. Med., 22:436-440;1925.

144. Papanicolaou,G.N. J. Lab and Clin. Med (Suppl) 75:79; 1941.

145. Papnicolaou),G.N. Science, 95:438-439; 1942.

146. Pauchet's Monograph: Quoted by "Symposium on Hormonal Cytology". 12:91; 1968.

147. Peters, H.: Acta Cytol. 4:146 – 148 and 153-154, 1960.

148. Phyllis, A., Cassano, C.T., Patricia, F., Saigo and Steven,I. Hadju: Acta Cytol 30: 93-98; 1986.

149. Pinto, RM., Viggiano C.H., Zunino NB., Videla E.A. and del Castillo E.B. Acta Cytol 12: 75-77; 1968.

150. Prunti, F.T.G.,: Britmed J. (ii), 615; 1956.

151. Pundal J.P. and Van Meensel, F.: Massonet cie, Paris, 1951 PP102.

152. Pundal J.P.: Acta Cytol 12: 101; 1968.

153. Pundal J.P.: Acta Cytol 12: 122; 1968.

154. Pundal J.P.: Acta Cytol 12: 124; 1968.

155. Pundal J.P.: Acta Cytol 3: 253–255 – 1959.

156. Pundal J.P.: Acta Cytol. 2:241–243 – 1958.

157. Pundal, J.P.: Acta Clin.Belg.5:66–71;1950

158. Pundal J.P.: Paris, Masson, et cie 1957.

159. Pundal JP and Liehtfus CJP, Acta Cytol; 3: 247–253; 1959.

160. Pundal, J.P.: Faris: Masson et Cie, 1966.

161. Pundal, JP., Acta Cytol 3: 211; 213, 219, 1959.

162. Pundal,J.P.(1952)Quoted by "Exfoliative Cytology in Gyanecological Practice" 2nd Edition Butterworth and Co. 1969,. pp80 London.

163. Ramos,M.G.:Acta.Cytol.3:298;1959.

164. Randel, C.L., Buetz, R.W. Hall, D.W. and Birtch P.K. Am.J. Obstet. Gynec; 69:643;1958.

165. Rehman D. and Zaman H.: Acta Cytol 7: 287-291; 1963.

166. Rizvi R., Khan, Ansar, A. and Khan, M.: Ind J. Pathol, Microbiol-page 165–170; 1978.

167. Rombaldi, R.L., Serafini, E.P., s Mandelli, J. et al, Vial J. 5:106; 2008.

168. Rokoff, A.E.: Acta Cytol 5: 153–167, 1961.

169. Rubenstein B.B. and Duncan, D.R. – Endocrinology 27: 843–856; 1940.

170. Rubertein, B.B. and Bendick, T: Nationals Research Council, 1942.

171. Rubio, C.A. Haules, S., Pareja, A., Acta Cytol 11: 176-178; 1967.

172. Rubio, CA: Acta Cytol 17: 361–365, 1973.

173. Ruiz, M.L. Acta.Cytol., 12:95–96, 101, 102, 113, 114–115;1968.

174. Ruiz, M.L., Maligna Cientiz, Medica, Barcelona; 1964, pp92

175. Schmitt, A. (1953) Quoted by Sonek 1967.

176. a. Saraiya, U. and Garud,M.A; J. Obstet. & Gynec. India;Vol xx1x : pp 837–842 ; 1979.

    b. Saraiya , U., Carvalho,B. andMehtaji, S: J. Obstet. and Gynec. India ,Vol. XXV1, pp.569–572, 1976.

    c. Savaiya., U.,: Proceeding of the Indian Academy of Cytologist. pp 30–33; 1969.

177. Sen. D.K and Langley, F.A.: Acta Cytol 16: 116-119; 1972.

178. Shamim J. Sami, Khan Ansar,A., Rizvi,R.; J. Obstet. Gynaee. India Vol XXVII; 158–1977.

179. Shearman, R.T. and Garret, W.J; Brit. Med.J., 1:292;1963

180. Shorr, E; Journal of Mt. Sinai. Hosp.12:667-688;1945

181. Shorr, E., Science: 94: 37 and 579, 1940.

182. Shorr,E. Science: 94: 545; 1941.

183. Sarkola, M.F., Grenman, S.E., Rintala, M.A. et al Acta Obstet. Gynecol. Scand. 87:1181–11; 2008.

184. Smith, O.W., and Smith, G.Van. S.,: Am J. Obst and Gynee 51: 411;1946.

185. Smith, O.W., Smith, G.V.S., and Schiller, S., Clin. Endocrinol.1:461; 1941

186. Smith, G.V.S., SMITH, O.W. and Pundal, J.P., Am. J. Obstet. Gynec., 399:405;1940.

187. Smolk,H. and Soost,J.J.; (1956) Quoted by Von Haam 1961pp326.

188. Soloway, H.B.: Acta Cytol 13: 136–138, 1969.

189. Struthers, R.A.: Brit. Med. J., 1:1331–1335, 1956.

190. Sonek, M.,: Acta Cytologica, 11:41–44; 1967.

191. Sora, M.,: Acta Cytologica, 11:41–44; 1959.

192. Soule, S.D.,: Acta Cytol 8: 368–372, 1964.

193. Spira, H., and MacRac, D.J.: J. Obstet. Gynaec. Brit Cwlth, 67: 597–607 : 1960.

194. Stieve,H., (1925, 1927),QuotedbyButtlerand Taylor,1973;pp239

195. Stone, D.F., Sedlis, E.D.A. Stone, M.L. and Turkel, W.V. Acta Cytol.,S 11: 349; 1967.

196. Stienhoff, R. (1965) Quoted by Ortner, etal.1977,pp429.

197. Struthers, R.A., Brit.Med.J; 1: 1331–1335;1956.

198. Symposium on Cancer cytology during Pregnancy; Acta. Cytol.3:41;1959.

199. Symposium on Hormonal Cytology, Acta .Cytol. 12: 87-127, 1968.

200. Symposium,on "Effect of Endogenous oestrogen" Acta Cytol 4:13 – 50, 1960.

201. Talwar, G.P. and Segal, S.J. Proc. US Nat Acad Science, 50;226–230; 1963.

202. Terminology Symposium. Acta Cytol 2: 63 – 139; 1958.

203. Terzano, G: Acta Cytol; 12 : 103; 1968

204. Terzano, G: Acta Cytol; 12 : 106; 1968.

205. Teter,J.Acta.Cytol.12:107;1968

206. Teter, J. Acta Cytol 12 :114–115 ; 1968.

207. Teter, J., and Boczkowski, K; Acta. Cytol., 11:449–455;1967.

208. Toth, F. and Gimes, G.: Acta morph Acad. Sci. Ung. 14 : 65–71;1966.

209. Tichy, M., Dyhora, H. and Havranek, J; Histochem. Cytochem.21–49;1964.

210. Tozzini, R., Sabrino, A.J., and Hoovis, E Acta Cytol 15: 57–63; 1971.

211. Ulfeder, H. and Meigs, J.B.: New England J. med., 237: 45–56; 1947.

212. Valenzuela, P., Sabatel, R.M., Valls V, Nieto, A. Gonzalez – Gomez, F., Int. J. Gynaecol Obstet 43 : 313-316; 1993.

213. Van Meensel, F; Bull. Fed. Soc. Gynec. et. Obstet. 49: 241, 1950.

214. Vedela, E.A. and DelCastillo, E.B.: Acta Cytol 13: 534–535, 1969.

215. Vital Statistic of United States, 1964, Vol II, mortality part-B.

216. Von – Haam,E. Acta Cytol 5: 320–329; 1961.

217. Von-Haam ,E. and T.D. Efstation: Acta Cycol 3: 209; 1959.

218. Wachtel E. Acta Cytol 10 : 56–61; 1966.

219. Wachtel, E.: Exfoliative cytology in Gynaecological Practice: 1969 2nd Edition Butter worth and Co, London.

220. Wachtel.: E. Acta Cytol, 2: 103 : 1968.

221. Watchtel E ad Plester, J.A.: Jobtel, gynace, Brit. Emp. 59: 323; 1952.

222. Wachstein, M and Meisels, E; Am. J. Clin. Path.; 27:13;–20;1957.

223. Wahi, P.N.: Seminar on Exfoliative Cytology organised by ICMR, N. Delhi–1969.

224. Weber E: 1972 Quoted by Ortner 1977.

225. Weid, G.L. Accta cytological, 8:383–384, 1964.

226. Weid, G.L. and Davis ME: Ann. N.Y Acad Sci, 83: 207–216;1959.

227. Wawryk,R,, Dudkiewicz, J.and Kubicka., A; Ginek. Pol.41:395-400;1970.

228. Weid, G.L; J.R. del Sol, and A.M. Dargan : Am. J. Obstet and Gynec., 75 : 98-111&289-300; 1958.

229. Weid, G.L.Am J.Obst.& Gynaec 70:51-59 1955.

230. Weid G.L; Am.J.Cl.Path 25:742-750 ;1955.

231. Weid, G.L., Obst. & Gynec., 9;646; 1957.

232. Weid G.L., (1953 Quoted by Ferin,J;1968 Pp 117.

233. Weid, G.L.,W& W.Christiansen; Quoted by Pundal p219;1959

234. Wisniowska, A. and Wierstakow, B. Ginek Pol. 43 : 421 – 427; 1972.

235. Wisniowska, A.: Akad. Med. Lodz (Thesis) 1970.

236. Willis, J., & Harley, J. M.G.,Brit.Med. J.,Feb. 12:399-401;1966

237. Wood, C. Osmond – Clarke, F., and Murray, M. J Obst Gynaec Brit Cwlth, 68: 778-1961.

238. Youssef, A.F. and Fayad M.M. J. Obstet gynec Brit comm. 70: 32–8;1963.

239. Zhuang Zuo; Goel, S. and Carter J.E. Am J. Clin Path, 136 : 260–265; 2011.

240. Zidovsky,J., – Monography Brathislava: SAV 1964.

241. Zidovsky, J.,Acta. Cytol;5:393–39;1961.

242. Zander,J., Acta Cytol; 3:197;1959.

243. Zidovsky, J. Vedra B., Mares, J., Horska, S., Edited by Horska, J and Stembera, Z. P291. Excerpta Medical, Foundation, Amsterdam 1967.

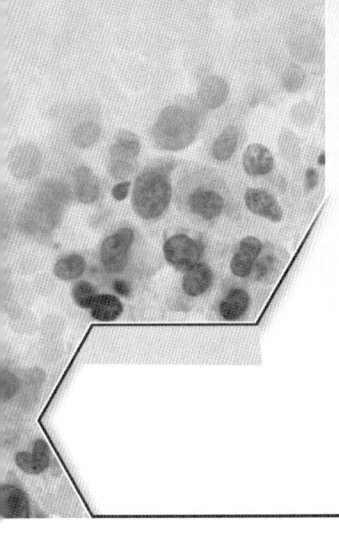

Index